The General Practice Journey

The future of educational management in primary care

T0133912

Edited by

Tim Swanwick

Director of Postgraduate General Practice Education
London Deanery

and

Neil Jackson

Dean of Postgraduate General Practice Education
London Deanery

Radcliffe Medical Press

Radcliffe Medical Press Ltd
18 Marcham Road
Abingdon
Oxon OX14 1AA
United Kingdom

www.radcliffe-oxford.com
The Radcliffe Medical Press electronic catalogue and online ordering facility.
Direct sales to anywhere in the world.

British Library Cataloguing in Publication Data

A catalogue record for this book is available from the British Library.

ISBN 1 85775 809 9

Typeset by Aarontype Ltd, Easton, Bristol
Printed and bound by TJ International Ltd, Padstow, Cornwall

Contents

Foreword

'I'm all for progress – it's change I can't stand.' This quotation sums up the feelings of so many general practitioners (GPs) about their professional lives. Just when you think you have mastered the latest plans for the development of the National Health Service (NHS), everything changes yet again. Whether it is the internal market, the abolition of the internal market, the end of fundholding, the appearance of foundation hospitals and trusts, or whatever next week's policy turns out to be, many doctors feel that they have become pawns in a political game, undervalued, and ignored.

But some things do, and indeed must, remain constant. As Bob Dylan, an academic not often quoted in the medical literature, once said, 'The more everything changes, the more it stays the same'. It is the absolute responsibility of those who work in the world of general practice education to ensure that the things that really do matter are the things that do remain unchanged. When the consulting room door closes, and the patient is alone with the doctor, the overwhelming importance of trust, safety, and clinical competence must remain – whatever the structure of the organisation that the doctor is working in.

The last few years have been characterised by dreadful problems with general practice morale, and consequent major workforce problems. The weekly medical press has portrayed GPs as being downtrodden, exhausted, demoralised, and undervalued. The powerful negative cognitive therapy effect that this has had on GPs leads to overwhelming negativity being transmitted to medical students and young doctors – hardly a recipe for solving the workforce problems that so bedevil us.

But in many cases, it is not the work that doctors feel stressed by, it is the job. Over and over again in recent months I have spoken at conferences and meetings where the vast majority of the audiences of GPs have said that they actually truly enjoy their work with patients. Julian Tudor Hart once described general practice as 'the medicine of patients with names' and this unique personal relationship between doctor and patient still seems to be of great value to both parties. Repeatedly over the last 12 months, general practice has been shown to have remarkably high approval and trust ratings – 91% in a study commissioned by the Cabinet Office – and it is essential that the changes that face general practice are not allowed to damage this powerful and therapeutic relationship.

Our working lives are going to change beyond recognition. The information explosion, skill mix, the breaking down of the primary and secondary care divide, the new contract, the changing demographics of both doctors and patients – all of these will have an impact. For generations, professions have been defined by the body of knowledge that they hold. When all the knowledge in the world is available via a computer costing under five hundred pounds along with a modem, the role of the professions must become much more that of advocate, mentor, guide, and support. After all, we will be no more effective at stopping change than King Canute was at stopping the waves. Whilst it has become a dreadful cliché to state that problems are only opportunities in disguise, it is nonetheless true – even if sometimes it feels as if we are surrounded by insurmountable 'opportunities'.

This book is a tremendously welcome addition to the literature of general practice education. While the threats are real, the opportunities for us all are truly remarkable. I believe that the next few years have the potential to deliver a renaissance of British general practice as profound as the changes of the 1950s and 60s – changes that resulted from the formation of the Royal College of General Practitioners (RCGP), and the charter that revitalised general practice in the sixties. Understanding the issues that face us is the first step – and this book clearly, concisely, and very readably summarises the story so far. The 'general practice journey' still has a very long way to go.

David Haslam
Chairman, Royal College of General Practitioners
July 2003

About the authors

The editors

Tim Swanwick MA (CANTAB) DRCOG DCH MRCGP
Tim has a broad range of experience in general practice education having been a trainer, and both an undergraduate and primary care tutor. Currently a Director of Postgraduate General Practice Education in the London Deanery, Tim is also a member of the panel of examiners of the Royal College of General Practitioners, sits on the editorial board of *Education for Primary Care* and writes widely on all aspects of general practice education and training.

Neil Jackson FRCGP DRCOG DFFP ILTM
Neil first entered general practice in 1974 as a full time principal and quickly developed an interest in education and training. He is a former GP Trainer, Course Organiser and Associate Regional Adviser in General Practice. Currently Dean of Postgraduate General Practice Education in the London Deanery and Honorary Reader in General Practice/Primary Care at Queen Mary College (Barts/Royal London Hospitals). He is a former MRCGP examiner and the author of various books, book chapters, peer-referenced papers and articles on general practice/primary care/education and training issues.

The contributors

Tareq Abouharb
Associate Director for new GPs
London Deanery

Reed Bowden
Associate Director
London Deanery

Paul Bowie
Associate Adviser
West of Scotland Deanery

Isobel Bowler
Project Manager
London Deanery

Charles Easmon
Regional Director
Workforce Development for London

Karen Finlay
General Practitioner, Tunbridge Wells
Course Organiser and APD Facilitator

David Haslam
Chairman
Royal College of General Practitioners

Anne Hastie
Director of Postgraduate General Practice Education
London Deanery

Sean Hilton
Professor of General Practice
St George's Hospital Medical School

John Howard
Associate Director
Mersey Deanery

Kevin Hurrell
Course Organiser
KSS Deanery Senior Registrar Scheme

Neil Jackson
Dean of Postgraduate General Practice Education
London Deanery

Peter Jenkins
Deputy Dean
KSS Deanery

John McKay
Associate Adviser
West of Scotland Deanery

Suzanne Savage
Associate Director
London Deanery

John Schofield
Associate Director
London Deanery

Vicky Souster
Educational Consultant
South London Organisation of Vocational Training Schemes

Dame Lesley Southgate
President
Royal College of General Practitioners

Tim Swanwick
Director of Postgraduate General Practice Education
London Deanery

Alex Trompetas
Associate Director
London Deanery

Rebecca Viney
Associate Director for GP Non-principals
London Deanery

Stewart Wilkie
Higher Professional Fellow
West of Scotland Deanery

Abbreviations

AD	associate director (or dean)
APD	accredited professional development (programme)
AUDGP	Association of University Departments of General Practice
BMA	British Medical Association
CME	continuing medical education
COGPED	Committee of General Practice Education Directors
COPMED	Committee of Postgraduate Medical Deans
CPD	continuing professional development
CPP	Committee on Professional Performance
CRAGPIE	Conference of Regional Advisers in General Practice
DEN	doctor's educational need
DHSC	directorate of health and social care
DPGPE	director (or dean) of postgraduate general practice education
EMQ	extended matching question
EU	European Union
GMC	General Medical Council
GMS	General Medical Services
GP	general practitioner
GPC	General Practitioners' Committee
GPR	general practitioner registrar
HA	health authority
HEI	Higher Education Institution
HCHS	Hospital and Community Health Services
HImP	health improvement programme
HPE	higher professional education
HR	human resources
ICT	information and communications technology
IM&T	information management and technology
IP	internet protocol
ISDN	integrated services digital network
ISP	internet service provider
JCPTGP	Joint Committee on Postgraduate Training for General Practice
KSS	Kent, Surrey and Sussex (Deanery)
LATS	London Academic Training Scheme
LIZEI	London Initiatives Zone Educational Incentives
LMC	local medical committee
LSG	local support group
MADEL	Medical and Dental Education Levy

MCQ	multiple choice question
MCU	multipoint control unit
MDO	medical defence organisation
MEQ	modified essay question
MPET	multiprofessional education and training
MRCGP	Member of the Royal College of General Practitioners
NAPCE	National Association of Primary Care Educators
NCAA	National Clinical Assessment Authority
NMET	Non-Medical Education and Training
NSF	National Service Framework
PACT	prescribing analysis and cost
PBL	problem-based learning
PC	personal computer
PCG	primary care group
PCO	primary care organisation
PCRN	primary care research network
PCT	primary care trust
PDP	personal development plan
PG	postgraduate
PGEA	Postgraduate Education Allowance
PGMC	Postgraduate Medical Centre
PGME	postgraduate medical education
PMETB	Postgraduate Medical Education and Training Board
PMS	personal medical services
PPD	personal and professional development
PRHO	pre-registration house officer
PUN	patient's unmet need
RAE	Research Assessment Exercise
RCGP	Royal College of General Practitioners
RHA	regional health authority
ScHARR	School of Health and Related Research
SEA	significant event analysis
SGPR	senior GP registrar
SHO	senior house officer
SIFT	Service Increment for Teaching
SLOVTS	South London Organisation of Vocational Training Schemes
UG	undergraduate
UKCEA	United Kingdom Conference of Educational Advisers in General Practice
UKCRA	United Kingdom Conference of Regional Advisers
VPN	virtual private network
VTA	vocationally trained associate
VTS	vocational training scheme
WDC	workforce development confederations

CHAPTER 1

Current concerns in the educational management of general practice

Tim Swanwick

The current agenda for the management of general practice education is huge and all-embracing and departments of postgraduate general practice education (deaneries), in addition to managing a burgeoning core business, are working in a highly complex and dynamic world. Nothing stays still for long in the NHS and the pace of change is faster than ever before. New relationships are constantly having to be forged, new lines of accountability developed and funding streams channelled, managed and merged. New ways of working are emerging all the time, with the constant development of new models of healthcare provision. As a result, questions are being asked of our existing training structures and also of the roles of GP educators and deaneries. Are they truly fit for purpose, and what should that purpose be? All this, plus mounting governmental pressure to respond to workforce demands in the face of a demoralised profession. It becomes no easy task then to both keep the ship afloat, and make headway through what are increasingly choppy waters.

The core business of departments of postgraduate general practice has traditionally been the management of vocational training with some overseeing of the continuing professional development (CPD) of GPs. But there is considerably more to it than that, as this book serves to illustrate. In the final chapter we shall look at some of the areas of new business for the providers of GP education and possible directions and futures for the UK deaneries. In the meantime, with primary care trusts (PCTs), strategic health authorities and the workforce development confederations (WDCs) on a steep learning curve, the National Clinical Assessment Authority (NCAA) taking its first faltering steps, and the Postgraduate Medical Education and Training Board in embryonic form, deaneries remain in the words of TS Eliot, 'At the still point of the turning world'.[1]

The United Kingdom Conference of Educational Advisers in General Practice (UKCEA) provides an annual forum for representatives from all the UK deaneries to meet and share best practice. In 2002, the conference was held in London, a location that encapsulates the complexity and pressures currently faced by these organisations. The London Deanery serves around 4000 GPs and manages 27 vocational training schemes and over 400 trainers. This results in an output of more than 300 new GPs each year. Deanery funding is held by five separate WDCs and the deanery relates, for the purposes of CPD, to 32 PCTs in very different stages of organisational development. There is an acute shortage of healthcare workers at all levels in London and a considerable lack of permanence. London in effect trains, at least in part, for the benefit of the rest of the country. London also has specific educational needs relating to its large ethnic and refugee populations. It is not surprising then that many of the concerns voiced in this book – recruitment, retention, performance and tapping into refugee and overseas doctors, to name just a few – have already been brought into sharp focus in London. Indeed, several of the chapters in this book are written by members of the London Deanery team.

The theme of the 2002 UKCEA conference was that of an odyssey. Not specifically Homer's epic wanderings, but what the *Collins English Dictionary* refers to as 'any long and eventful journey'. The journey for general practice, certainly an eventful one, takes us from undergraduate education through vocational training and from there into the emerging envelope of higher professional education (HPE) and onto the lifelong learning arena of continuing professional development with its newly wrought links with public accountability and performance management.

All stages of the 'general practice journey' were visited during the conference and our book is based on keynote speeches and workshops undertaken there. There were many more workshops than we have prepared chapters but these selected highlights provide a fascinating and informative cross section of deanery activity at the present time. Where possible, workshop members have been credited for their contributions.

But enough pre-amble, I encourage you to embark on the *General Practice Journey*. Read on, but bear in mind that in postgraduate education, our world today will have changed by tomorrow. Points of departure will have shifted, directions of travel altered and the staging posts along our journey relocated. Ultimately though, it is this constant flux that keeps us engaged and interested – a process of iterative rediscovery succinctly celebrated by Eliot in his *Four Quartets* – and in wishing you bon voyage, I leave you in the poet's company again:

> We shall not cease from exploration
> And the end of all our exploring
> Will be to arrive where we started
> And know the place for the first time.[1]

Reference

Eliot TS (1963) Four Quartets in *Collected Poems 1909–1962*. Faber, London.

CHAPTER 2

The interface between undergraduate and postgraduate general practice education

Sean Hilton

Keynote speech delivered at the 2002 UKCEA conference

It is a great pleasure to be invited to give this presentation at what I believe to be an exciting time for collaboration between undergraduate (UG) and postgraduate (PG) wings of GP education. When I first took steps from full-time general practice into academic practice fifteen years ago I think it would be fair to say that relations between the two wings were sometimes distant, and in some cases antagonistic. There were historical explanations for this, but in recent years we have seen many more reasons for partnership and collaborative working. In my view, the latest changes to the structure and organisation of the NHS give us opportunities to strengthen further our collaborative approach.

In this presentation, with respect to the interface between UG and PG GP education, I would like to spend some time covering:

- where we were, where we are now, and where we might be going in UG education
- how might we integrate UG and PG education, what might we integrate, and why?

Where we were

Thirty years ago, I was a medical student, and in my three years of clinical training I spent not one hour in general practice – my future career.

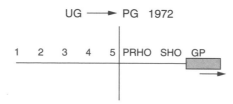

Figure 2.1 Undergraduate to postgraduate experience of general practice in 1972.

This disconnection between UG education and eventual career, as illustrated in Figure 2.1, was quite striking, particularly on one's first day entering general practice!

At St George's Hospital Medical School in recent years, when we were making the case for establishing an accelerated graduate entry scheme for primary medical degrees, we made great play of the following quotation (possibly apocryphal, but attributed to Sir Henry Barcroft of St Thomas' Hospital):

> The study of medicine is a useful way to pass the time until the student is mature enough to become a doctor.

I am not sure of its vintage, but certainly there was little obvious link between what we did, particularly in the first two years of the course, and what happened to us once we qualified.

Moving forward 20 years to about the time when I became head of the UG department, general practice had made some inroads in the curriculum. Figure 2.2 shows a typical pattern of attachment at that time.

There would be a short block of time in the third or fourth year – perhaps a fortnight – and then some attachment in the final year. Often students would disappear around the country and fix up some time to spend with a GP. There remained a long gap between qualification and exposure to general practice. Nevertheless, we had advanced quite a way, and around this time Justin Allen and colleagues published their discussion paper on academic general practice.[1] The authors, representing both sides of 'the divide', argued that academic general practice had come a long way in the preceding 20 years, but could achieve a lot more with shared resources and management structures. It was, perhaps,

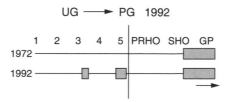

Figure 2.2 Undergraduate to postgraduate experience of general practice in 1992.

optimistic for the time, but made some convincing arguments about some of the problems that were arising because of the artificial separation. These were:

- it was difficult to establish research, with a lack of output and influence on central research policy
- because we were split, academic credibility could not be established easily
- difficulties in recruitment
- a low overall contribution to academic medicine (less than 1% of GPs enter academic posts versus 5–10% in many specialities)
- overlapping roles in education and training leading to duplication of efforts.

From that time I have seen much greater enthusiasm for tackling the problems, and I do believe that over the last seven or eight years we have had some success.

Also highlighted in that article was the lack of career structure for academic general practice. In 1993 the Association of University Departments of General Practice (AUDGP) did publish proposals on career structure – Figure 2.3 was at the heart of it – in which we attempted to set out a progression for young GPs to work though to senior status.[2]

The details are less important than the principles, but even so there were a number of problems with it, that we recognised clearly in the text of the report. Firstly, most people (myself included) had entered from the side of this career track, quite some way down the line. This was still happening – and still does today – and it was neither possible nor desirable to discourage this route. Secondly, it was not easy (although we made suggestions) to map closely onto that figure a similar progression through the stages of PG GP education through to regional adviser as the equivalent to professor. Nevertheless, the report helped

Years since qualification	Title	Time distribution	
		Clinical %	Academic %
1	PRHO	100	0
2–3	SHO	100	0
4–5	Academic trainee in general practice	50	50
6–9	Associate academic GP/lecturer	50	50
10+	Senior lecturer	35	65
15+	Professor	20	80

Figure 2.3   A proposed career structure for academic general practice (AUDGP 1993).

us to think carefully about the issues. In recent years we have had productive annual meetings between the United Kingdom Conference of Regional Advisers (UKCRA) and AUDGP (before we both changed our names!) and publications. I believe positive changes in approach and attitudes have come from these.

Where we are now

So where are we now, with UG medical education, in terms of our structures, opportunities and activities?

We have made significant progress in UG education in general practice over the past 10 years, and the blocks of GP exposure now are much more prominent (Figure 2.4).

This has really occurred in the curriculum reforms that followed publication of the General Medical Council's (GMC's) document *Tomorrow's Doctors* in 1993.[3] Typically, there is now early clinical exposure in years 1 and 2, and predominantly that is in general practice. It is about meeting patients with chronic disease, learning about the impact of illness on patients and their families, and often 'family studies' where students follow pregnant mothers through late pregnancy and after the birth of the baby. It is also about learning clinical and communications skills more formally and intensively. So we have a greater component of the curriculum overall, of the order of 10–15% of time, compared to the 2–3% given to us in the past. We also have pre-registration house officer (PRHO) posts in general practice, although not in great numbers, and the opportunity to focus more on the senior house officer (SHO) grade appointment as part of the general review of early PG training, about which you will be more informed than me.

Thus a long way has been travelled in the past 10 years. So much so that as heads of department in UG schools we felt it time that we revisited the *Mackenzie Report*, work published in 1986, predominantly by John Howie and David Hannay, recording the contributions made by general practice departments to medical schools in the UK.[4] It was both a census of activity in departments at that time, and a consideration of the challenges facing them. The Mackenzie II

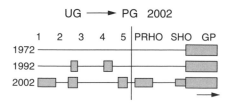

Figure 2.4   Typical general practice experience for undergraduates in 2002.

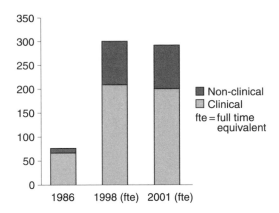

Figure 2.5   The growth in numbers of staff in academic departments.

report, entitled *New Century, New Challenges*, will be published in Autumn 2002.[5] The following are extracts from that report. It is instructive to compare the establishment and activity of the departments over the 15 year period, though interestingly the challenges are much the same.

In 1986 there certainly was not an academic department in every university medical school. There has been since 1992, and by the time we ran a census in 1998 the numbers had peaked at just below 300 (*see* Figure 2.5). The substantial increase in non-clinical members of staff is predominantly on the research side but not exclusively. Although 1998–2001 was a time of rapid expansion in GP teaching activity, there was actually a slight fall in numbers, and this reflects a squeeze in funding within the higher education sector. Thus there has been a substantial increase in activity, not matched by increased staff numbers, and that is causing some difficulties. Examining that in more detail, in 1986 a student in their undergraduate career would typically experience 20–40 GP sessions in five years, approximately 2–3% of the clinical curriculum. There were approximately 2200 practices nationally taking students on attachments. Departments had minimal involvement in schools' central organisation of curriculum or examinations. In 2001, the activity had nearly trebled (mean sessions in general practice in UK medical schools 120, range 80–132), so that on average we are delivering around 9% of curriculum time, and a higher proportion of clinical attachment time, around 15%. This still may sound like an inappropriately small proportion of the total, but it does illustrate how in the past the effects of a single 2–3 week spell in general practice would be obliterated by the remainder of the time spent in secondary or tertiary care.

The number of practices accepting students has risen markedly to approximately 3600 practices, and continues to grow, and I will come back to this issue later. Also now there is a prominent involvement of GPs in the central organisation of curricula and examinations.

The range of activity for UG teaching is now much wider, including:

- early clinical contact
- communication skills
- clinical skills
- specialist 'firms'
- 'integrated learning week'
- primary care attachments
- special study modules.

I have already mentioned early clinical contact, and the evaluations of that are positive, showing it to be very much valued and appreciated by students. I feel that it demonstrates right from the start that general practice is an important part of their future careers. Very often, as most of you will know, we are strongly involved in the clinical and communications skills teaching; and in some cases specialist firms, such as medicine, or cancer care, are established. One of the developments is in the graduate entry programme at St George's, a four year course for graduates in any discipline. Every week during the first two years of that course, the students have a 'problem of the week', which acts as the focus for the learning of their problem-based learning (PBL) curriculum. They have a session in general practice each week, with a patient suffering from a condition relevant to the 'problem of the week' be it, for example, hearing loss, angina or infertility. The session with their GP tutor thus represents a key part of their learning week, and their learning is grounded in a clinical case discussed with their GP tutor. The more traditional general practice/primary care attachments are still occurring in increasing numbers, and there are additional opportunities such as special study modules – areas of student-selected study in depth. Thus students are learning more about clinical medicine than by 'sitting with Nelly' that formed our only teaching opportunities in the past. They are learning about the practice of medicine in the context of general practice.

Turning to research, although there is a long history of outstanding individual GPs as researchers, from Edward Jenner through to Mackenzie, Pickles and Fry, I personally have always felt that research is a much less natural activity for us as GPs than is education. The nature of our daily clinical work is inductive rather than deductive. Nevertheless, strong research in general practice is very important in order to broaden its academic base (as opposed to simply broadening the base of academic general practice). UG departments, predominantly in the shape of individuals, have made major contributions to spreading research throughout general practice. I do feel we need to build on that, and not simply focus on departments. *The National Report on R&D in Primary Care*, led by David Mant,[6] and the MRC's *Topic Review of Primary Care*,[7] led by Nigel Stott, have helped to set the agenda for primary care research, not only in the nature of the research priorities, but also in the structures. The primary care research networks (PCRNs), now running successfully in most regions, arose from that work, and are generating research in general practice that needs to be supported and nurtured by UG and PG departments.

Data from the *New Century, New Challenges* report show that of over 900 research staff and students in the UK departments of general practice, the highest proportion is for MSc students (approximately 40%). I feel that is a very important contribution to generating the research culture in general practice that we need.[5] Clinical researchers comprise only around 15%, with non-clinical research staff making up approximately 25%, and the remainder being MD or PhD students.

Looking at the areas of challenge identified in this report, they split really into three:

1 challenges for academic GPs – about maintaining and attempting to lead clinical excellence when we have to spend a lot of time out of clinical practice
2 career progression challenges are still there (with accreditation, re-accreditation and clinical governance issues coming up, these challenges are even greater)
3 challenges for departments within medical schools. Even though they are essential to educate the next generation of doctors, it is important to strive for excellence in research because that is such a fundamental part of funding support for medical schools. There is a dilemma between meeting the demands of the Research Assessment Exercise (RAE), which is about international excellence and long-term programmes, and the demands of NHS research which is often about applicability, local relevance and short-term results. This causes difficulties for medical schools as well as departments, in how they use their limited resources. Then there are the wider NHS challenges that we also need to be contributing to.

Kendrick and Smith surveyed heads of departments and directors of postgraduate general practice education during 2001 to establish the levels of current collaborations.[8] The area where most was happening was in joint teacher training or practice approval. Other frequent collaborations include the shared use of IT facilities, or shared use of simulated patients from a bank or resource. There was also a lot of activity on developing PRHO posts, and joint extended training schemes following vocational training is another key. Rather more initiatives are planned but not yet under way. Some PG members with university appointments do some joint teaching in assessment of general practitioner registrars (GPRs) and in masters degree teaching that I have already alluded to, and there is a range of other schemes.

In terms of the benefits from collaboration, essentially these are educational and intellectual benefits; perhaps we work more effectively together in promoting general practice as a career; collaboration also generates opportunities for capacity building and building and expanding networks, and economies of scale.

I wanted to take this opportunity to mention a scheme close to my heart, which is LATS (invoking memories of boy scout camps in childhood!), because it is a good example of an extended vocational training initiative, and one on which we have some good evaluation.[9] LATS was the 'London Academic Training Scheme', which was led by Professor George Freeman from Imperial School of Medicine, and it arose from the LIZEI era (London Initiatives Zone Educational Incentives scheme). The scheme enabled the funding of a number of one year training posts. There were a number of aims and objectives for LATS posts (*see* Box), but note those highlighted in bold type.

Registrars were encouraged to develop a research project that would be presented to the peer group. This created a supportive pan-London group of LATS registrars working together on day release courses to modify and carry out a range of self-generated research projects. On the teaching side they had opportunities to experience one-to-one and small group teaching (including multidisciplinary groups). To gain some familiarity with inner city practice there was a clinical commitment of three sessions per week, and opportunity to see how that kind of work might link with academic general practice. The numbers entering

---

London Academic Training Scheme (LATS)

Aims and objectives
By participating in LATS, registrars will be able to:

- **overview the research process**
- discern soluble and relevant research questions
- undertake a focused literature review
- be aware of quantitative and qualitative research designs
- **present a research idea to peer group and expert, and then modify the plan**
- know where to find and how to use expert help
- **experience one-to-one and small group teaching, including multidisciplinary groups**
- design, complete and begin to disseminate his/her own research project
- **gain familiarity with inner-city practice and how this can link with an academic department**
- **make an informed choice about personal involvement with academic general practice.**

the scheme topped 50 by the time the LIZEI funding came to an end. Sadly this was before the Medical and Dental Education Levy (MADEL) transfer of vocational training funds came through, and so we were unable to apply to keep it going in the ways we would have liked to. There are now new opportunities arising with senior GPR appointments, and we remain optimistic about reviving the scheme. However, 55 registrars went through the original scheme within the five participating London medical schools. Looking at the outcome, we were able to survey all of the registrars in years 1–4 of the scheme, 49 of them, and we received full replies from 32. It is heartening that all but two of them were still working in general practice. The two had switched to public health training. The large majority were working in London, and just over half retained attachments to or appointments in academic departments. Of those in departments, two-thirds held research posts, and one-third had specific teaching posts.

Finally in this section on where we are now, it is worth noting from a geographical perspective how the opportunities have grown for interaction between UG and PG general practice educators. Figure 2.6 shows how medical schools in England and Wales were only five years ago. We were in a fairly stable situation. The only really changing scene at that time was all the medical school mergers taking place in London, where over a period of years we went down from 12 independent schools to five – one in each health sector of the capital. Otherwise, the schools of the UK were well established, and there were

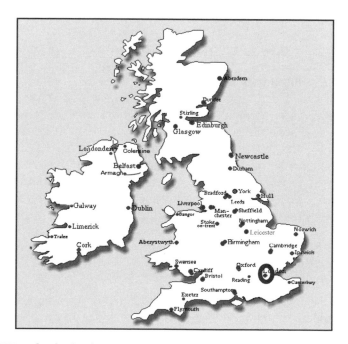

Figure 2.6   UK medical schools 1997.

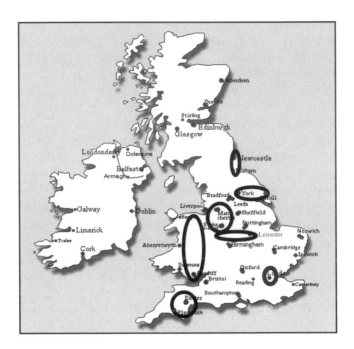

Figure 2.7   UK medical schools 2003.

corners of England and Wales with very little activity from general practice undergraduate education. Figure 2.7 shows the expansions of UG schools following the large increases in medical student numbers. All of those 'corners' are now covered. Not only have the student numbers gone up everywhere, but also areas in the north east, in the east riding of Yorkshire (York/Hull), East Anglia (Norwich), Midlands (Keele/Manchester, and Leicester/Warwick), south west (Peninsula Medical School) and south east (Brighton/Sussex) all have new medical schools or campuses. In Wales, UWCM Cardiff has spread, so that its clinical attachments have become very much 'pan-Wales'.

So, geographically all the bases are covered, given that the overall numbers of UG students will be rising over three years by 40% – from an annual intake of approximately 5000 to 7000. The number quoted above of 3600 practices taking medical students on attachment will rise further.

Where we might be going

My track record on predictions is not good, so in turbulent times such as these you would have to put wide confidence intervals on my opinions – many things might happen in the next five years. (One possible future is depicted in Figure 2.8.)

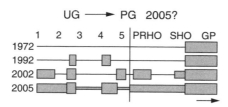

Figure 2.8 Undergraduate to postgraduate experience of general practice in 2005?

I am not sure how much further we will go. **I am** sure that we will have further representation within the standard five year curriculum. The new medical schools all seem to have substantial general practice experience planned for their students from year one. I believe that we will increase the PRHO GP provision, but there is a good deal of work still to be done on this. The role of general practice experience in the general professional training of junior SHOs should be clarified in the coming years, and it looks likely that general practice experience will form an important part of it. My message is that the small block of general practice time in 1992 (*see* Figure 2.2) is gradually transforming into a solid longitudinal line of experience of general practice that commences early in the MB.BS course and continues throughout UG and early PG training. To provide this, we need a shared approach, and shared resources. I believe the latest structural changes to the NHS and the funding of education and training within it do provide some opportunities for us (*see* Box).

The merging of the NHS education and training levies, SIFT (Service Increment for Teaching), MADEL, and NMET (Non-Medical Education and Training), is a significant step, particularly when taken in conjunction with the new more localised management of the funds by the newly created WDCs. This change is all happening at the moment, and it is early days to see whether its effect will be to advantage or disadvantage attempts to work in an integrated way. However,

---

Opportunities for shared approaches and shared resources

Multiprofessional Education and Training (MPET) levy managed by WDCs

- **not** MADEL versus SIFT versus NMET

Information and communications technology (ICT)

- evidence-based medicine online
- distance learning
- web-based learning

taking one example – and I referred to PRHO posts in general practice earlier – if we look constructively at the PRHO year as being the final year of basic medical training, it may be helpful in supporting the supervision workload that is something of an issue in expanding these posts further.

Then there is ICT, on which I am certainly not an expert, but I do believe that this will change education radically. It can only be to our advantage to work together in harnessing this. Distance learning and web-based learning are very important to us within the medical schools as I am sure they are for PG general practice education.

Undergraduate–postgraduate integration – how, what and why?

How?

It would be wrong to deny that there are obstacles to our increased collaboration, even for those of us that are committed to it. For one thing there is the sheer pressure that is induced by workload and short-term priorities. Secondly university and NHS demands are not always compatible, and I have referred to how this can cause difficulties in research. Nevertheless I feel the NHS structural changes already referred to have helped rather than hindered. One year ago in our sector of London, my opposite number in PG general practice education, held a joint meeting between our departments to discuss how we could collaborate fruitfully under new arrangements. There are four areas where we felt this to be particularly promising:

- PCT/strategic health authority liaison
- post-vocational training opportunities
- educational staff development
- research.

For example, the new PCT agenda is such a large one, and under such pressure, that we felt there was little room for us to be trying to work separately, when we could be working in a concerted way with PCTs to help them, and to also utilise opportunities that they will be able to provide for us. There are enormous challenges, but a motivated GP workforce is something that is essential to the survival of the NHS. It is not something that we can provide on our own, but we are able to make a contribution through the education, support and stimulation that we can offer. The multiprofessional education agenda is also a huge challenge and, for the moment, it is a very high government priority so there is much encouragement for us to develop this. How are we to address the agenda, and still make education stimulating and exciting as opposed to another task that must be done to deliver the latest set of requirements? This is not easy – but as challenges that we face together, I believe we can tackle them more successfully together.

What?

In terms of our shared educational business, Simon Smail and I argued in a paper published last year that we are moving towards a position where we can define a lifelong curriculum, that begins in the earliest stages of medical school and continues through to retirement.[10]

We can plan this together, and deliver it together. I would like to start at the end that concerns me more closely at the moment, and summarise what happens in our St George's curriculum. If you are more familiar with other medical school curricula you will probably find a similar approach. That is, as well as having blocks (modules) of teaching and attachments, there are 'themes', 'strands', 'spines' or 'threads' that run longitudinally through curricula from start to finish.

In fact, we have two separate curricula, but they share the same four 'themes'. We happen to organise them in this way, but it is the principle rather than the detail that is important. We base our content and approach around **basic and clinical sciences; patient and doctor** (predominantly clinical and communications skills); **community and population health** (which is more or less self explanatory, but we aim to ensure that those perspectives are prominent in students' experience); and **personal and professional development** (PPD) – exceptionally important areas for those going on to a career as medical professionals. To some extent all of those themes are present in general practice exposure, but you can envisage there are some where general practice has a greater contribution to make than others. Simon and I suggested the following as being particularly suitable for the general practice lifelong curriculum:

- critical appraisal
- ethics and law
- PBL/problem solving
- consultation, communication and clinical skills
- IT skills
- clinical governance.

At St George's these are predominantly handled within the PPD theme, but that is less important than the fact that they are recognised as important

---

What is distinct about general practice?

- Community and population perspective
- Natural history/long-term nature of disease
- Long-term nature of doctor–patient relationship
- Patient involvement and motivation
- Multiprofessional teamwork
- Informatics in health

---

components at all stages of development. All are essential for good clinical practice in primary care. This may be self-evident to us, but my feeling is that if we are explicit about it to students they will appreciate it more readily. We know that there are many things on looking back whose importance was far from clear to us at the time, and I feel we can do better in this regard with today's medical students.

These major components of lifelong learning are relevant to general practice, but they are also important in all branches of medical practice. So what is there within them that is distinct about general practice, and that we can start viewing from the earliest stages? These are shown in the Box.

The involvement of patients and their motivation, plus multiprofessional learning are areas where we are already well placed to provide this, more so than with hospital-based care at the present time.

Why?

To me this whole area feels a little like asthma management in the late 1980s and early 1990s. At that time we felt we were improving our management year on year, and yet the secular trends in prevalence and severity of asthma were moving so fast that we had difficulty in keeping pace with them. Similarly the pace of change, initiatives, demands and target setting is such that it is very difficult to keep pace with the demands for education and training. If we work effectively together (as primary and secondary care finally began to do with asthma management) we should make better progress – not that we can solve the problems of the NHS, but together we can make important contributions to its continued success.

It seems to me that there are several factors that really threaten general practice as we know and value it. Promotion of the lifelong curriculum for general practice is needed to help us counter this. These factors will be familiar to all of you in the difficult environment in which we work:

- public perceptions
- GP morale
- structural/contractual changes
- 'generation X'.

Generation X is my shorthand for a concern that I have heard from colleagues in all branches of medicine about why current PRHO, SHO and registrar grades have values that differ from those that we were prepared to enter the profession with. Values such as partnership, commitment, on-call, 'going the extra mile' are not there as they used to be. People are more assertive and demanding in what they expect from us. That is a real challenge – to see the world through the eyes of those that have different values from us, who may feel committed to general practice but not in the ways that we have felt. I feel we can do better from the very beginning to address these issues, and define, encourage and support professional development that is appropriate for the future state of general practice.

Summary

I believe we have come a long way in the past 30 years to make general practice – and the values and skills that it promulgates – indispensable to the UG medical curriculum. Now we must utilise the opportunity that we have created to pass on better prepared graduates to the PG training phase. The new NHS structures and funding streams do give further opportunities even though they are complex and difficult. In this presentation I have referred to a lifelong curriculum for general practice, and I see this as the centrepiece in which presently constituted undergraduate and postgraduate departments of general practice can work more closely together. In the NHS there is a pressing need for workforce development that we both tap into. We must seek to deliver what is wanted by the NHS for its prosperity – a committed and motivated current and future workforce for general practice and primary care.

References

1   Allen J, Wilson A, Fraser R and Pereira Gray D (1993) The academic base for general practice: the case for change. *BMJ.* **307**: 719–23.

2   Association of University Departments of General Practice (1993) *A Proposed Career Structure for Academic General Practice.* AUDGP, Oxford.

3   General Medical Council (1993) *Tomorrow's Doctors. Recommendations on undergraduate education.* GMC, London.

4 Howie J, Hannay D and Stevenson J (1986) *The Mackenzie Report – General Practice in Medical Schools of the United Kingdom – 1986.* Macdonald, Edinburgh.

5 SAPC (2002) *New Century, New Challenges. A report from the Heads of Departments of General Practice and Primary Care in Medical Schools in the UK.* The Society for Academic Primary Care, Liverpool.

6 NHS Executive (1997) *National Working Group on R&D in Primary Care: final report.* Department of Health, London.

7 Medical Research Council (1997) *Primary Health Care (topic review).* MRC, London.

8 Kendrick A and Smith F (2001) Survey of heads of department and directors of postgraduate general practice education. Unpublished survey.

9 Freeman G, Fuller J, Hilton S and Smith F (2001) Academic training in London. In: J Harrison and T van Zwanenberg (eds) *GP Tomorrow* (2e). Radcliffe Medical Press, Oxford.

10 Hilton S and Smail S (2001) A lifelong curriculum for general practice. *Educ Gen Pract.* **12**: 1–10.

CHAPTER 3

Creating relevant SHO posts for general practice training

Vicky Souster and Suzanne J Savage

Traditional hospital posts for vocational training scheme (VTS) doctors are sometimes unsuitable but how can they be improved? What makes a good post 'work' educationally? Is moving the location from hospital to community likely to solve all the problems? A research project conducted by the South London Organisation of Vocational Training Schemes (SLOVTS) has uncovered some 'keys to success', which we would like to share. We also have first hand experience of pitfalls to avoid.

The aims of this chapter are to:

- use the SLOVTS experience to demonstrate how innovative posts may be funded, set up and integrated into current local educational initiatives
- discuss the findings of the SLOVTS research project, and its implications for successful innovation in GP education
- encourage those involved in VTS management that new initiatives, if well managed, can dramatically improve the learning experience of doctors.

Setting up innovative posts

The SLOVTS was set up using Tomlinson funding in 1994, and has been funded since by the health authority and PCTs in inner South East London. This has unlocked funding to support innovative community-based training posts, which are not managed by the local trust hospitals. SLOVTS has employed support staff to improve the management of the posts, including an education consultant. She has supported course organisers by implementing educational developments and conducting evaluation and research. The popularity of the

SLOVTS innovative posts has had a major impact on the number of GPs applying for VTSs in inner South East London. Because of increased competition for places the SHOs entering the schemes are of an exceptionally high standard.

The term 'innovative' indicates that the SLOVTS-managed posts differ from 'normal' VTS training posts in three main ways:

- at least half of the training is situated in the community rather than an acute hospital setting
- some of the staff supervising the training are specialist nurses and other professionals
- the funding for the posts is provided by the PCTs in Lambeth, Southwark and Lewisham, enabling SHOs to be supernumerary in all or part of the posts.

The research project was conducted because innovative posts had been running for 5–8 years. Initial evaluations by course organisers who had set up the posts were very positive, but it was felt that a rigorous qualitative research project was now needed to assess the factors that had improved the learning experience for SHOs. One post from each of the three schemes (based at King's, Lewisham, and Guy's and St Thomas' hospitals) was selected for the study to give a variety of specialities and settings. The research explored the post from the perspective of the educational supervisors, senior nurses, and course organisers, to ascertain their roles and their effect on the educational experience. A summary of interviewees is shown below.

King's 'women's health' post	SHO on VTS × 2	Clinical specialists × 2	Course organiser × 1	Community midwife × 1
Guy's and St Thomas' 'homeless, rootless, drug addicted' post	SHO on VTS × 2	Clinical specialists × 2	Course organiser × 1	Clinical nurse specialist × 1
Lewisham University Hospital 'community mental health' post	SHO on VTS × 2	Clinical specialist × 1	Course organiser × 1	Senior community psychiatric nurse × 1

In all three posts, two VTS doctors were interviewed who had completed training in the specialist post within the last 12 months, giving a total of six SHO experiences. Four of the six doctors who gave feedback about the SHO posts were registrars in general practice at the time of interview, as they had reached their final year of training. They were able to make judgements about the effectiveness of their training in the light of their experience as GP registrars.

The interviews were tape recorded and transcribed prior to independent analysis by both researchers, and key themes were identified. The main author then rejected themes that were not regarded as significant by both researchers, and disregarded any themes that had little or no evidence to support them from the interview data. The interview schedules were designed to test whether barriers to learning reported in the literature (1990–2001) had been removed, and to explore other key factors that have created a positive environment for learning.

Literature review: barriers to learning for SHOs on vocational training schemes

- Core skills needed for general practice (whether generic or subject specific) were not identified.[1]
- Appropriate learning opportunities within hospital settings were not utilised.
- The acquisition of appropriate skills and knowledge was not demonstrated by the end of the training.[1]
- SHOs were undertaking non-medical tasks.[2]
- No educational targets had been identified.[2]
- Appraisal of performance was not done.[2]
- SHOs felt unsupported in coping with work-related stress.[2]
- No regular assessment of progress took place for 67% of SHOs on VTSs in hospital posts. These results were from a large-sample questionnaire survey of all SHOs in VTSs (including the armed services) in the UK on 1 April 1989. The response rate was 73%. Of those who did have an assessment, some reported that it was not until the end of the post, or that the results were not shared with them.[3]
- Only 27% of 165 SHOs in the Trent region VTS reported having a formative assessment.[4]
- Most of the 161 consultants in the Trent region who were training VTS SHOs said that there were educational objectives for the post, but only 29% of the SHOs reported their use in practice. This revealed a gap between the intentions and educational practice of consultants.[4]
- Hospital consultants have no protected time for delivering education: if they use time allocated to clinical work then they have to justify the lower productivity of their department to NHS managers. They are also not paid for any educational time they give (unlike GP trainers and course organisers) and pressures on their time can seriously affect the quality of the educational experience for VTS individuals and other SHOs.[5]
- Grant and Marsden[6] have described the 'creation of a climate for learning' as the key aim for educationalists, where work takes place in an atmosphere

of openness and SHOs participate in their learning by actively seeking information. In their study they identified that the fear of 'not knowing' and consequently of being judged as a failure, militates against the formation of an ideal learning environment. The authors suggested that there is a clash of needs when junior doctors are responsible for patient care. The patient needs reassurance and decisive action, and the SHO needs advice, support and supervision. If the latter are not available, learning opportunities will be missed, and SHOs may fail to become confident in their skills.

- Styles drew an analogy between abusive family systems and medical education.[7] He suggested that in both there are 'unrealistic expectations, indirect communication, the denial of problems, and a system in which the learners feel isolated. Negative judgement and blame are common and direct feedback with positive suggestions for improvement are rare'.
- Positive supervision is a critical component of effective education. Where trainers convey their belief that learning involves continual support and advice to learners a 'climate for improved learning' will prevail.[6]

The published peer-reviewed literature revealed a lack of in-depth interview studies that explored VTS posts. None of the studies had examined SHO posts in the community. This study is unusual because it has collected data from SHOs, course organisers, nurses and clinical specialists, and explored the relationships between them.

Key research findings

The site of the learning experience

All of the posts were originally redesigned because it was felt that acute hospital experience was unsuitable for a GP training post. The alternatives found in the three different jobs varied enormously in terms of the experience that they offered. Clinical experience included:

- outpatients clinics serving the community, e.g. family planning, sexual health, community midwives clinic
- specialist treatment centres, e.g. a community detoxification unit, a specialist addiction clinic in the community
- a hostel for homeless men
- a walk-in mental health advice service.

SHOs working in the innovative posts felt that they were much more relevant to their future role as a GP.

I got to see normal patients which is maybe a bit more relevant to the future, and it was just a good chance to examine an awful lot of people and it was so nice ... to suddenly get out into the community and see people who had normal blood pressures and you know everything was going right for a change rather than everyone you saw on the sort of wards where it was all going wrong. (SHO 5)

I think lots and lots of hospital jobs, psychiatry hospital jobs and paediatric hospital jobs, you're doing things that ... you aren't going to ever use again, you know I'm never going to have to hold somebody down and give them rapid tranquillisation ... as a GP. ... It's not something I am going to be using day to day, and I just think that the community post that we had was much more relevant to general practice and psychiatry. (SHO 1)

Many other clinical experiences could be accessed for visits or short periods. These were usually observation periods, whereas in the main components of the experience SHOs were expected to take clinical responsibility for the patients. The most positive learning outcomes were associated with the higher levels of responsibility for patient care, which SHOs reported as a major change from hospital work:

I: What have you particularly enjoyed about this training post?
R: Gosh. I think so many things. It was the ... partly I suppose it was the independence, and for the first time really, the experience of being a doctor, on your own, making decisions ... you really feel like you make a difference, which I'd never experienced before, having only worked in hospital. (SHO 4)

Provision of appropriate support and supervision for learners

Good quality supervision (where provided) enabled the SHOs to learn from their clinical experience in a very productive way. However, the siting of posts in the community did not guarantee that SHOs would be supported, and in some cases lack of support caused problems and a less than ideal training environment.

I think initially I felt quite unsettled because I was moving from place to place with the job, and I did find it a bit difficult, especially if I was trying to ring a GP, for example, if I was just kept on hold for, for a long time. So I think from a practical point of view it was often difficult to ask for help.

I never felt like I couldn't ask for help, it was just often if you were being held for ten minutes, you just find it a bit frustrating. (SHO 3)

In contrast, other sites provided excellent supervision so that skills could be built up gradually:

We limit the amount of patients they see, we give them as much time as they need. They're always supported, they're never left alone in this particular bit of the job. (educational supervisor 2)

The quality of support and supervision is a major factor in the success of a post, and one danger of community posts is that people move around a lot or are based in different sites on different days of the week. In one case this entailed SHOs working without direct supervision, and this in turn resulted in a lack of feedback about progress:

I: And were you able to act upon the comments you received if you got feedback about your performance?

R: It was ... it was difficult because you are essentially an independent body. No-one's there to see or supervise you or see your progress. It's only ... I mean it's based very much upon what you feed back to your supervisor. So I mean I was able to act on, on most of what was fed back to me, but in the same instance it wasn't supervised, nobody saw my progress, and no other person fed back to, to the supervisors as regards how I'd been progressing, so ...

I: So how did the supervisor know how you'd been progressing? Was it on your personal ... how you reported it?

R: I mean it's ... I guess it's from ... I mean it's how I fed back to him. I mean in addition I think it ... I think they usually get to hear about it through nurses or you know, other staff and things if, if people aren't happy with the doctor.

The situation highlighted above was obviously not providing optimum learning, and the course organiser rearranged this part of the post as soon as the research findings were shared.

The course organisers and educational supervisors interviewed stressed the importance of working with other professionals as part of the learning experience. This is very important in the general practice environment but not always a feature in SHO hospital posts. The SHO interviewed below clearly appreciated both the emotional support given by the nursing team, and also the learning to be gained by review and reflection:

There was constant informal feedback, because you were going through clinical cases the whole time. I mean every Monday when we had a meeting, you know, you'd be talking about clinical cases. You know, once a week we're meeting with one of the specialist nurses who's going through those sort of things and, and they're very aware; more, more aware than any post I've ever been in of what, what's actually going on with people. And have to be, 'cos quite often personal issues come into these, these things ... you know, if you're consulting with people who have a lot of emotional problems ... you've got to also be aware of your own emotional state. (SHO 4)

Articulation of aims and learning outcomes

The most successful innovative posts had established clear aims and learning outcomes. Without these the SHOs were in danger of becoming passive observers rather than active learners. The community setting felt very alien if the SHOs were used to hospital medicine and they needed clear guidance about the clinical responsibilities that they were expected to take on, and the levels of specialist knowledge needed to support their clinical work. In posts where this was established at the beginning, the SHOs felt safe enough to take clinical responsibility, providing there was adequate support and supervision available.

The posts where the aims and learning outcomes were clearly articulated were also the most successful in terms of providing a positive learning experience. This was because the objectives were not static, but were set and reset during the training period. This facilitated continuous review of both the education and the clinical experience provided. In one such setting the course organiser felt that the appropriateness of the training was due to his attending formative assessment meetings.

I would do a formative assessment at two months and four months, and ... there was a very clear sense that at the four month assessment, you know, it was a building on and from the two month, that there'd been a sense of progress ... you know, new learning objectives had been formed or learning objectives had been modified and there was a sense of progress there. (course organiser 2)

He maintained this commitment for the first two years that the post was running and then withdrew. According to the SHOs interviewed, the education supervisor had maintained the quality of training since then without course organiser input. In other posts input by course organisers was needed to maintain standards, but they had withdrawn at a point when everything was going well.

Complex posts caused problems for SHOs if they did not have clear explanations about their roles and responsibilities. They also need guidance about the level of knowledge they were expected to attain. Learning objectives formulated by the Royal College of General Practitioners (RCGP) with a traditional hospital post in mind did not 'fit' the community-based post.

> I found it quite difficult to sort of get into the various bits of the job, because I didn't have anything definitive in front of me to say, 'Well this is what you should be taking away, or this is what you should know in order to ... in order to carry out the various aspects of the job that you're doing.' (SHO 3)

The quality of the SHO's experience was adversely affected by lack of communication between SHOs, course organisers and consultants/specialist nurses, because feedback about the training experience was lost.

Access to resources that support learning

Grant and Marsden identified the provision of resources to support learning as an important factor for SHOs in training.[6] Interviewees in each setting were asked about the provision of resources such as books, CDs, models, videos, and planned teaching sessions. In fact the SHOs and course organisers identified people in the clinical setting as the most important resource. The specialist nurses, who managed one of the units, were the first point of access if SHOs needed information, and team meetings were used to explore clinical dilemmas. The provision of planned teaching varied in each post, and between posts, but there seemed to be a correlation between length of time spent in a specialist area, the provision of GP-orientated resources, and SHO confidence in the subject. Those that moved swiftly through many short-term experiences seemed less satisfied with their learning experience, and were less positive about the usefulness of the post.

Course organisers were not involved in advising educational supervisors about teaching tools such as books that would be relevant for SHOs. Tutorials and other teaching events were highly valued by SHOs, but in some posts the SHOs missed learning opportunities because they were simply not aware of them. This seemed to be the result of poor educational organisation (for example a secretary had lost the timetable), or due to a misunderstanding by the educational supervisor, who assumed that SHOs on the VTS would not want to attend a teaching event planned for specialist SHOs.

Some SHOs did not have learning resources available. One educational supervisor admitted that he was not an expert in the area that he supervised, and did not know where further resources to support learning could be accessed. Another problem was the loss of teaching resources since the post was set up, such as clinical sessions with experts who had dropped out of the programme because of changes to working patterns and personnel. In one case an interesting aspect of the post was lost when a consultant died, and the clinical experience had not been replaced. The original vision for some posts (which was exciting and positive) was not in fact being delivered due to such changes, but course organisers were not requesting clear formal feedback from SHOs, so were unaware of this.

Information provided at induction varied from post to post. One consultant provided a comprehensive pack including all basic reading materials, patient information leaflets, timetables, a job description and relevant articles from journals. This was the only site where there were teaching materials specifically geared towards GP training. Another post had an on-site specialist library and computer aided learning packages, and the third post had a major university library on-site. SHOs did not, however, access the libraries to a great degree; most of them relied on the working knowledge of others in the clinical situation. Some of the learning support was very imaginative, for instance SHOs in one setting attended a specialist conference with the consultant, which they found extremely useful.

Communication between learners and key staff involved in the VTS

The three course organisers interviewed had little knowledge about the working practices of educational leaders within the post, and they assumed that clinical supervision and assessments were still happening as had been planned when the post had been set up.

> I think it is fair to say that if a job is running well, then the course organisers don't tend to look in too great a detail. I mean they check and say, 'How's it going?' and they'll check and say, 'Is everything okay, and do you feel properly supported?' and all that sort of stuff and the guy's saying, 'Yes, yes. It's wonderful, it's wonderful, it's wonderful'. Then the ... I'm afraid the course organisers have got other things to do and therefore they all tend to say, 'Well thank goodness for that'. And I guess that's why I'm feeling particularly I need ... we need to sit down and review the post so that I can feel more confident about what I think is going on. (course organiser 1)

In fact, some of the educational supervisors (clinical specialists) were unsure what was expected of them, and were confused about their supervisory responsibilities. None of them were in regular contact with a course organiser.

> I don't think I've ever seen printed educational objectives ... I don't think I've ever read them, or I don't have a copy. What I do is to sit down with the

VTS SHOs and decide well what – you know, given that this is the design of the post, what would you particularly like to get out of it? So it's individualised rather than general, but I think there are some generic ones somewhere. (educational supervisor 3)

The lack of clarity and poor communication can be attributed to several organisational factors.

- Training was taking place in more than one site, so supervision was split between clinical leaders in different sites, and also the specialist nurses. The SHOs in these situations did not know who to relate to as their primary supervisor.
- There were no regular planned meetings or communication between supervisors in different elements of the post and course organiser for that post.
- Changes in personnel had occurred, and when educational supervisors left, the course organisers made assumptions that new staff would behave in the same way as their predecessor. This was rarely the case.
- There was lack of awareness about the supervision provided, due to a lack of formal feedback mechanisms. Course organisers were unaware of cases where supervision and assessment had not been provided for SHOs.

Discussion

This study has revealed many of the processes that both enhance and detract from SHO education in VTSs. The burden of service provision had been reduced for these SHOs, enabling them to learn more and be more self-directed. However supervision, formative assessment and appraisal were not necessarily better managed in these posts. The role of the specialist nurses as supervisors is both complex and ambiguous. They have no contact with course organisers, and although SHOs clearly appreciated the emotional support that the nurses gave, they did not acknowledge their role as teachers in the clinical setting.

Having clear aims and learning outcomes is important if the value of time in each post is to be maximised. Where there are several strands of clinical experience, each needs to interface with the others, and this can only be achieved if the educational leaders (both specialists and GPs) communicate regularly.

It was unfortunate that all of the course organisers interviewed had become progressively less involved with the innovative posts. Course organisers in this study did not appreciate how much the clinical specialists needed them for advice and support. The need for course organisers to maintain the clarity of aims and objectives in each part of the post, and monitor the quality of supervision has been clearly demonstrated by this study.

Many of the less desirable aspects of training were not recognised (or not acknowledged) by those providing the training, but this was not because SHOs were afraid to highlight problems. SHOs were actively communicating with various people involved in the management of the post, but a lack of formal evaluation and communication prevented the message from reaching the people who could act upon it. There were no regular reviews of the posts in this study: these would have provided a time and place where problems could be discussed and successes celebrated.

Conclusion and recommendations

This study demonstrates that educational success was linked to three educational strategies: case review and discussion as teaching methods, effective clinical, emotional and educational support for learners, and clear ideas about what was to be gained from the training post. Enabling SHOs to take responsibility for patient care through good clinical supervision is the key to a satisfying learning experience, and provides them with the confidence to manage specific clinical problems in future. Follow-up of patients is also important, so that the outcomes of clinical decisions are learnt about.

Formal assessment structures added little to the SHOs' learning experience unless they were carried out by clinicians who worked in close proximity to the SHOs, and who could give accurate feedback about their performance and progress. Clear aims and learning outcomes could be adapted for each individual SHO, but this needed a facilitator who could help the SHO to transform the desired learning outcomes into his or her personal learning needs. This process is more likely to happen if the learning is planned, documented, and reviewed at formative assessments.[8]

As a result of the research project, SLOVTS has been able to identify a 'recipe for success' for those wishing to set up 'innovative posts' which seek to provide a more relevant training for GPs (*see* Box).[9]

Setting up and managing relevant SHO posts: the SLOVTS recipe for success

- Keep it simple: have one educational leader responsible for SHOs throughout the post, and one base site for the SHOs.
- Have regular reviews (at least annually) to reflect on SHO feedback. Major changes in educational provision may be needed, and course organisers need to be proactive in this area.

- Ensure that the staff engaged in educational supervision are providing what the SHOs need. Educational supervision should ideally be done by people who are interested in, and willing to engage in, GP training. If such a person leaves it cannot be assumed that their replacement will have the same standards and working practices.
- Ensure that quality remains high by evaluating, reviewing and (where necessary) re-shaping the post. Training posts are not static entities, and need to be actively managed to remain successful.

In the face of current and future GP shortages, strategies that attract young and able doctors into the primary care environment are vital. The formation of local WDCs may facilitate locality planning to deal with specific staff shortages and funding issues. Popular VTSs affect the quality of patient care both in the hospital and the community, and bring people into an area that they may not have considered otherwise. Innovative training schemes have the potential to make general practice training more relevant, more effective and more attractive as a career option.

References

1 Kearley K (1990) An evaluation of the hospital component of general practice vocational training. *Br J Gen Pract*. **40**: 409–14.

2 Rickenbach M (1994) Hospital vocational training – local audits are helpful [letter]. *BMJ*. **309**: 196.

3 Crawley H and Levin J (1990) Training for general practice: a national survey. *BMJ*. **300**: 911.

4 Baker M and Sprackling PD (1994) The educational component of senior house officer posts: differences in the perceptions of consultants and junior doctors. *Postgrad Med J*. **70**: 198–202.

5 Bayley TJ (1994) Commentary: the hospital component of vocational training for general practice. *BMJ*. **308**: 1339–40.

6 Grant J and Marsden P (1992) *Training Senior House Officers by Service Based Learning*. Joint Centre for Education in Medicine, London.

7 Styles William McN (1990) But now what? Some unresolved problems of training for general practice. *Br J Gen Pract*. **40**: 270–76.

8 COPMED (1995) *SHO training: tackling the issues, raising the standards*. A discussion paper by the Committee of Postgraduate Medical Deans (COPMED) and the UK Conference of Postgraduate Deans, Jan 1995.

9   Souster V and Marriott P *Organising Education to Create a Climate for Learning: a qualitative study of three innovative GP training posts in South East London*. Research report, SLOVTS. Unpublished.

The team at SLOVTS is happy to offer support and advice to other providers who wish to explore setting up innovative training posts. A full report of the research undertaken is available from SLOVTS. Contact SLOVTS via email (www.slovts.org.uk) or phone the team (+44 (0) 208 7922 8115).

CHAPTER 4

Recruitment and selection for general practice – sharing good practice

Isobel Bowler and Neil Jackson

Significant changes in the means of funding general practice training – the 'MADEL transfer' – were set out by the Department of Health in the *Health Service Circular 1999/230* (DOH, 1999) and implemented for English general practice training from April 2000.[1] In effect, funding for GP vocational training, including GP registrars' salaries, expenses and the trainers' grants, was transferred from the General Medical Services (GMS) budget to MADEL.

In Wales, a similar transfer of budgets occurred from April 2000. In Scotland, GP registrar salaries had already been transferred from health boards to the Scottish Council for Postgraduate Medical and Dental Education in April 1998, and in Northern Ireland the transfer of the GMS budget to the Northern Ireland Council of Postgraduate Medicine and Dental Education occurred in April 1999.

Following the 'MADEL transfer' directors, or deans, of postgraduate general practice education (DPGPEs) became the managers of the funding for GP training accountable to their PG deans. Along with this, DPGPEs assumed the responsibility for the recruitment of doctors to GP VTSs and GP training practices with an emphasis upon fair and open recruitment systems, rooted in appropriate equal opportunities for all applicants.

Since the inception of the 'MADEL transfer', deaneries in England have worked together through the Committee of General Practice Education Directors (COGPED) to develop deanery selection and recruitment procedures. Models of good practice and developmental progress have also been shared between DPGPEs from the four UK countries through COGPED. This collaborative approach has led, in England, to various initiatives including a co-ordinated national recruitment advertising campaign and clearing system managed through a national recruitment office.

The UKCEA workshop (June 2002)

Given the historical background described above, a number of workshop participants gathered together at the 2002 UKCEA conference to share their experiences of the general practice recruitment and selection process. A list of participants is given at the end of this chapter.

Sharing experiences

There was found to be a large degree of similarity in current selection procedures with all deaneries represented at the conference using assessment systems designed to test a set of competencies. The degree of centralisation of the process varied. A number of common elements emerged including comprehensive references used for short-listing. These were obtained by using a structured application form, with questions requiring written answers to assess competencies although difficulty was reported by some deaneries in obtaining completed forms from some referees.

The majority of deaneries were using centralised short-listing and ranking of candidates and two deaneries (Northern Ireland and Trent) were using a fully centralised interview process for all potential GPRs, but were processing small numbers within a compact deanery geographical area. Trent has developed an assessment centre approach, which uses structured interviews and observation of a number of assessment exercises e.g. role play of the doctor/patient consultation. Most other deaneries were using structured interviews, but had devolved these, to a greater or lesser extent, down to VTS level. Potential GPRs were interviewed by panels from the schemes they had applied to and many deaneries were using the 'same day same place' approach. Appointable GPRs not offered a place on a scheme of their choice could be seen straight away on another scheme.

A summary of selection and recruitment experiences shared by workshop participants is given in Table 4.1.

Issues and problems identified

In the summer of 2002, some deaneries were still having difficulty getting all assessors – notably some course organisers – to agree to a deanery-wide approach to appointing GPRs. There was also progress to be made towards a fair approach, conforming to good and legal practice, especially in terms of equal opportunities. Such compliance is essential and, illustratively, some deaneries reported that legal actions had already been taken against them.

Liaison with human resources (HR) departments varies and can be excellent. However, some participants reported difficulties in their relationship with trust

Table 4.1 Summary of selection/recruitment experiences as shared by workshop participants

Deanery	Centralised short-list	MCQs	MEQs/ structured written questions	Structured references	Structured interview	Centralised interviews
Manchester	•	•	•	•	•	Same place different panels
Wessex	•		•			•
Eastern	•		•	•	Working towards	Same place different panels
Wales	•		•	•	•	Same place different panels
Northern Ireland	•		•	•	•	•
Trent	•		•	•	•	• And other assessments
Kent, Surrey and Sussex (KSS)	• Long list by local panel		•	•		
Scotland			•	•		
Oxford			•	•		
Mersey	•		•	•	•	Same place different panels
London	•		•	•	•	Same place different panels

MCQ: multiple choice question.
MEQ: modified essay question.

HR departments. The issue of unappointable doctors remains a difficult situation to manage and there is a need to give good careers advice and support to these doctors. The workshop participants also discussed the issue of minimum standards, that is, what are they and how should they be assessed?

Next steps

Further goals in relation to good selection and recruitment practice and how these might be achieved were discussed. The total centralisation of recruitment by deaneries was not seen as desirable or achievable. However, it would be useful to maintain a national database of applicants, and where they are appointed. This would enable good quality data to be compiled nationally although there would be a need to comply with the Data Protection Act.

It was agreed that increasing the similarity of approach so that a GPR selected in one deanery would be appointable in another is desirable, and something to be aimed for.

Moving towards a similar approach

It was agreed by the workshop participants that the following areas would merit further development.

- A set of quality standards could be agreed and shared between deaneries possibly starting with the Trent competency framework. If this was evaluated it could form the basis of a national approach.
- An application form using open-ended structured questions to assess these competencies could be shared but a wide range of questions would be needed to select from to prevent model answers being produced.
- A shared structured reference form should be agreed.
- Short-listing criteria should be agreed. It was noted that this would entail agreeing a scoring system for application forms and references and assessors would need training in the same way to ensure similarity of approach.
- It was felt that the next phase i.e. the face-to-face element of the selection procedure would be more difficult to make uniform across deaneries.
- More research was needed to help deaneries understand the effectiveness of different assessment methods.
- Possibly there is some role for a national recruitment office but it was felt that applications should still be handled by deaneries.

Reference

1   Field S, Allen K, Jackson N *et al.* (2000) Vocational training for general practice in England and Wales: the dawn of a new era? *Educ Gen Pract.* **11**: 3–8.

Based on a workshop given at the 2002 UKCEA conference. With thanks to the workshop participants Isobel Bowler, Drs Alan Carr, Kevin Hill, Agnes McKnight, David Gibson, Simon Smail, Steve Lazar, Andy Hall, Barry Lewis, David McKinlay, Ian Mclean, John Howard, Neil Jackson.

CHAPTER 5

Crisis, what crisis? GP recruitment and retention – the RCGP view

Dame Lesley Southgate

Keynote speech delivered at the 2002 UKCEA conference

One of the things that I want to do is to reflect on the whole issue of 'what crisis' both from my perspective as President of the RCGP and from my own personal perspective. I want to consider whether there is a crisis, and if so what form it takes and what we can do about it from within the profession.

Problems in workforce planning often arise because solutions are proposed by individuals outside medicine, who do not always understand the underlying issues.

Is there a crisis?

Much of what I am going to say is based on the newly published seventh report of the British Medical Association (BMA) cohort study of 1995 medical graduates,[1] which seems to highlight some of the relevant issues. This is a 10 year longitudinal study of the career paths of about 545 doctors; it provides information on workforce participation, career choice and views about practising medicine.

Career choice

The seventh report shows that about 34% of respondents still want to enter general practice, which is greater than the proportion who said that they would choose general practice when they graduated. Thus there has been a shift towards general practice over the years, but this is insufficient to sustain the general practice workforce, which is estimated to be 55%. The numbers in the study are of course very small but can perhaps be accepted, for the sake of argument, as indicating that we do not have enough people choosing the discipline to replace those leaving. Also important is the fact that 65% of those choosing general practice are women.

What are graduates doing now?

Seven years after graduation, many doctors are working outside the traditional training and career structure: they are off seeing the world, experimenting with different work patterns and delaying settling down. Over a half of GP respondents had worked as locums during one year and only 37% had worked as principals: why should this be?

It is useful to consider some quotations from the BMA report from different people who have different levels of motivation to continue working in medicine.

Quotation 1 – strong motivation to medicine

My desire to practise medicine has increased in the last year. This is largely due to an extended period working outside the NHS. I have used medicine as a means to travel, I have worked in the private sector and I am now working in the Australian Health Service. All of these organisations have a different approach to management to the NHS but they also treat me very differently.

Quotation 2 – strong motivation to medicine

I have more autonomy in making clinical decisions, I have much better senior support when needed, I am learning a lot more and am working significantly fewer hours per week. I am not expected to work overtime routinely. If we are short of doctors for whatever reason, extra people are brought in. In short I no longer feel taken for granted. As a result, I am enjoying my job again and think, as a result, I am much more productive and a better doctor. I was planning a one year trip to Australia but am now considering staying for longer. Because of all my ties I am keen to return home but do not think I will return to the NHS.

More autonomy in making clinical decisions, much better support from seniors, learning a lot more, working significantly fewer hours – these are things that, in theory, we aspire to in training and in CPD, but I would argue that we are not quite delivering these aspirations.

Quotation 3 – lukewarm about medicine

I continue to find it very hard balancing career with family life. However, my present job has been created to fit in with school hours which is excellent. The downside is that my job is very quiet and on the research/outpatient side of medicine and not very fulfilling.

This quotation is from someone who has difficulty in balancing career and family life and is probably a woman. Is it not possible to create part-time jobs that are both family-friendly and professionally satisfying?

Quotation 4 – regrets about becoming a doctor

Undervalued, beleaguered, overworked. Often wonder why we bother.

There were quite a few similar comments in the report, much in keeping with the findings of a recent evaluation of PRHO placements in general practice.[2] Young hospital doctors, in particular, but also some GP trainees feel undervalued and left out.

What is the nature of the crisis?

I do believe that there is a crisis, and I think there are four contributing factors. The first is the difficulty, referred to above, that doctors have to try to combine work, family life and leisure time. The second contributing factor is the profound lack of understanding outside the medical profession as to how medical expertise is acquired. When we try to raise this issue, we are accused of being arrogant, of considering that we are brighter than everybody else, that we are worth more and that we should earn more money.

A third factor contributing to the crisis is the criticism and blame levelled at the medical profession over the last few years and which must be having a profound effect on the numbers of people applying to medical school. Unfortunately the volume of criticism is likely to increase, as, with insufficient new doctors, it is going to be difficult to deliver the *NHS Plan*. The effect of a culture of blame and criticism on the morale and motivation of staff has recently been explored in research undertaken by the King's Fund.[3] The research found poor morale and motivation to be a result of poor human resource practices that left staff feeling unvalued and unsupported. It was also linked to the perception of the profession. The research highlighted the gap between management rhetoric and continuing practice. For example, although there is talk of a 'learning culture' in the NHS, staff report that mistakes still result in the marginalisation and discipline of individuals.

Last, but not least, is the effect on morale of the undermining of generalism and the notion that somehow or another we are wasting our medical training by working as GPs. This undermining is absolutely fundamental in general practice, and is one of the reasons why we feel bad about life. There is a move towards a culture with fewer doctors per head of population, where doctors would be working in larger teams and where skill-mix would play an important role. But is that what the public wants? And how do we find out what they want? We are beginning to see a fragmentation of the doctor's role, which will be a serious problem for the development of the clinical generalist or medical generalist. More fragmentation and more specialism will lead to the acquisition of a different sort of expertise and loss of continuity of care. If the undermining of general practice continues we are going to start to compromise the benefits that other countries want to work towards. These benefits include high-quality care at a lower cost when compared with other types of healthcare systems.

Concomitant with the growing trend for the GP to be part of a large group of healthcare workers is the undermining of the GP's individuality, which can also have an effect on morale. Doctors' expertise is being disabled by having to work in dysfunctional systems – something we seem unable to explain to politicians.

How medical expertise is acquired

Findings from research on medical problem solving indicate that both novices and experts use hypothetico-deductive reasoning. The difference between experts and novices is in the details of the content and the organisation of medical knowledge. What is also important is the activation phase in experts: they go through a controlled deliberate processing phase in deciding what to do, what the diagnosis is and what one is going to do next. It is efficient, it is deliberate and it is expert.

How is this approach acquired? Findings from research on medical problem solving are again helpful in demonstrating that medical diagnostic expertise is content-specific and limited to clinical problems with which a doctor has substantial experience. It is the result of acquiring a body of knowledge, which is honed, expanded and organised through experience. This has major implications for teaching, learning and assessment and for maintaining morale and public confidence.

Seeing patients, reflecting on patients' problems and discussing each other's patients adds to our total knowledge and enhances problem-solving and diagnostic skills. Clinical practice is about individual experience with individual patients; about trying to fit the things that don't fit and adding to the range of things that need to be considered, and it is about completing the task, not hiving bits off to others.

If you are protocol- and guideline-driven the entire time and if you are externally reminded and controlled at the time, you don't develop the way you should. Experienced clinicians show great individuality of thinking and great individual effectiveness.

What can we do about the crisis from within the profession?

I have suggested four reasons for the crisis in recruiting and retaining young GPs; these have implications for teaching, learning and assessment and about the way we approach CPD.

Improve learning and assessment processes

I have argued that there is no substitute for clinical practice as a means of acquiring expertise in clinical medicine. Thus, important features of professional learning include clinical work and responsibility, backed up by close senior–trainee relationships and with feedback on performance, directed in such a way that people can change and develop. Feedback should be a routine part of work and a part of regular appraisal. Unfortunately, feedback is often inadequate or destructive, and assessment is of poor quality. This, combined with negative role models – demoralised, exhausted doctors with low esteem – contributes significantly to the crisis, with juniors thinking 'Why should I bother?'

Too much assessment of established doctors is process-based and irrelevant rather than outcome-based. Measures must relate to actual practice and the knowledge and skills that underpin it. Outcome **is** difficult to measure – it has to allow for the fact that doctors are individuals, they organise their knowledge in different ways, and they get to different end-points in different ways and at different speeds. But this does not means that we should not try to measure outcome. Subjecting established doctors to boring, trivial assessments can only lead to further demoralisation.

Features to consider in planning professional learning/assessment are summarised in the following Boxes.

Important features of professional learning

- work-based assessment
- appropriate role models
- induction into professional practice not studentship

Implications for assessment

- There is no reason to assess general problem-solving skills independent of medical content and context.
- Ability to apply (not just recall) knowledge and skills in clinical situations should be assessed.

Design of clinical assessments

- Problem-solving skills are content-specific and develop as a result of clinical experience.
- Performance in one clinical area does not predict performance in other areas very well.
- Specific problem areas and skills to be mastered should be identified and educational experiences that promote mastery designed.

It is important to remember that, in searching for meaningful outcome measures for measuring expertise, the expertise of teams can mask the lack of expertise in individuals. This, too, can have an important effect on morale if you know you have some dysfunctional members in the team and everybody else is going to have to cover up for them.

Improve working arrangements and relationships

In addition to boosting morale through changes in our CPD/assessment processes, we can attempt to make improvements to workload, personal style and partnership arrangements. We can even try to be nicer to each other! It is important to feel respected and valued by colleagues. We can try being there for each other and saying the right words when things aren't going very well, when somebody has had a really tough time on-call and wants to talk about it, or when somebody is feeling rather anxious about managing a patient and doesn't quite like to admit it; but some support and encouragement in the professional sense is fundamental to job enjoyment, particularly now, when many doctors feel they are often carrying out policies that do not fit with their personal values or are aware of a conflict of interest between providing service and increasing throughput and maintaining standards of practice.

Question current trends

I have referred to fragmentation of the GP's role, and some would argue that the concept of the GP specialist contributes to this. Most of the things that seem to be 'special interests' also seem to be core general practice. The RCGP is trying to work on this, though it has seen its role as developing a conceptual professional framework and guidance based on the interface between primary and secondary care and has been very careful not to stray into contractual areas.

But perhaps we doctors should be challenging the changes being forced upon us, and asking for evidence that they will improve healthcare or be more cost-effective. Thus, looking ahead, it is likely that nurse practitioners will replace GPs as a point of first contact in the main providers. Clinical nurse specialists will integrate hospital with community care for chronic disease; GPs will specialise in complex health problems, and care assistants will replace practice nurses, and that is fine. But is it what we want? Is it what the public wants? There is increasing evidence that developments in team working to date have been driven by policy not evidence and that the expected benefits are not always attained. Thus, quality of care is about the same with doctors and nurses, but there is no saving of GP time or NHS resources because nurses and counsellors work more slowly. The disbenefits have also been neglected – for example, the lack of continuity and co-ordination of care. How do we ask the public if this is what they want? My fantasy would be that a large proportion of people who can afford it would start seeking private or individual care with a GP or another doctor. I don't see a clamour in the private health sector for the kinds of multidisciplinary practices that are emerging in the public sector. Of course, perhaps the public don't know what is 'good' for them, they need educating on that and perhaps doctors have a role here. For those interested in influencing the future direction of general practice, the European definition of *General Practice and Family Medicine* is a good starting point.[4] Copies are available from the RCGP.

Conclusion

There is a crisis in recruitment and morale in general practice. This is due to the difficulty in balancing work and home life, a failure to understand how medical expertise is acquired, the undermining effect of criticism and blame, and the undermining of generalism that has accompanied the policy of team working. Measures the profession could take to improve matters include improving learning/assessment procedures for established doctors that measure outcome not process; improving our work arrangements and relationships; and questioning developments that undermine generalism and the individual effectiveness of experienced clinicians.

References

1   Lambert TW, Evans J and Goldacre MJ (2002) Recruitment of UK trained doctors into general practice: findings from national cohort studies. *Br J Gen Pract.* **52**: 364–72.

2   Grant J (2001) *Pre-registration Home Officer (PRHO) Placements in General Practice.* OUCEM, Milton Keynes.

3   Finlayson B (2002) *Counting Smiles: morale and motivation in the NHS.* King's Fund, London.

4   WONCA (Europe) (2002) *The European Definition of General Practice/Family Medicine.* WONCA (Europe), Trondheim.

CHAPTER 6

Increasing GP training capacity – sharing experiences

Suzanne Savage

Life is somewhat like when you are on a boat and there is a wind blowing. You cannot control the wind, but if you set your sails right, you can get to your destination.[1]

Increasing training capacity in order to increase GP numbers is and will remain a priority for deaneries, PCTs, WDCs and government. Training capacity is dependent on two components: hospital SHO posts recognised for GP training and GP-approved trainers and their training practices. To increase one without the other risks chaos. A personal enquiry was carried out to discover what stops GPs becoming trainers in the SE London sector, as a project completed by the author for her postgraduate certificate of education. A summary of the findings was presented to a workshop at the 2002 UKCEA conference and forms the basis of this chapter.

The 307 SE London sector practices were asked how training could be made more attractive. Six barriers to becoming a trainer were categorised. Triangulation of the results was possible by looking at other work done in this area. The enquiry produced a number of recommendations that could increase training capacity.

Method

A data collection tool was sent to all practices in SE London using health authority mailing lists. It asked GPs what was stopping them from becoming trainers and for any suggestions about what might make the role more attractive. Data

from primary care groups (PCGs) concerning manpower and trainers and training practices were collected and collated. Previous published work in this area
was analysed.

Results

In SE London there were no registrar vacancies in March 2002. Table 6.1
shows the numbers of doctors, practices, trainers, training practices and GP
vacancies in March 2002.

The table shows that the doctor workforce has more than 10% vacancies.
Existing trainers working at full capacity (assuming all trained doctors stayed
in SE London) cannot meet this shortfall.

Responses to data collection tool

Seventy-five written replies were received, the majority by email. Two of the
written responses were from trainers groups representing 20 trainers. Thirteen
responses were by phone calls (total response rate 106/848 (12.5%)).

Six barriers to training were identified. Figure 6.1 shows the proportions of
the six categories.

Lack of time

Half of the respondents were concerned about lack of time, both to train and to
be a trainer. '... my biggest problem is that to become a trainer, you need to
commit so much time.' (reply 1) 'I simply do not have the time to leave the sur-

Table 6.1 Numbers of doctors, practices, trainers, training practices and GP vacancies in
March 2002

PCT	Doctors	Practices	Trainers	Training practices	Doctor vacancies
Lambeth	170	55	15	9	7 (4%)
Southwark	171	61	12	6	26 (15%)
Lewisham	155	49	12	9	14 (9%)
Greenwich	102.5	49	10	7	11 (11%)
Bexley	92.38	37	7	5	16.6 (17%)
Bromley	158	56	11	9	12 (8%)
Total	848.88	307	67	45	86.6 (10.2%)

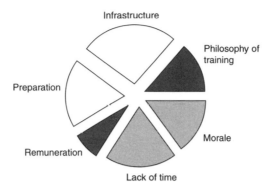

Figure 6.1 Barriers to becoming a trainer.

gery unattended.' (reply 51) 'Why I don't complete the training to become a trainer is because there is not enough time.' (reply 13)

There seemed to be a vicious cycle of not enough doctors causing practices to have no time to develop in other areas such as training. General practice was described as being '... so busy' (reply 74), with '... so many new imposed tasks'. (reply 33) 'I went on the first course a few years ago but have not carried it further due to the pressures of work in general practice.' (reply 57) 'If practices are working at near capacity it would be difficult to consider devoting time to being a trainer.' (reply 7) 'Protected time. This needs to be made a reality for training.' (reply 29) '... we used to occasionally go to the gym in between surgeries and we went home for lunch not too many years ago. Now we get to the practice at 08.30 and are rushing about like maniacs until 7 pm. I would be worrying continually that I had no time for the registrar.' (reply 64) 'Years ago it was felt a trainee was a help in the practice but I would see it as a hindrance as I would want to give a lot of time to the registrar to ensure they had good training and that is impossible now with the work load I have.' (reply 70)

Conflicting interests including UG teaching were mentioned as competing for time. 'I have taken on a lot of undergraduate training which I enjoy.' (reply 11)

Low morale of general practitioners

It was disturbing to find the contrast between those that said things such as a 'great job but too much of it' (reply 10), and those that were deeply unhappy with the job and had no enthusiasm to try to teach others about it as illustrated by comments such as: 'I wonder if GPs feel enthusiastic about training others for a role that a large number are unhappy with?' (reply 49) 'Sorry to sound so "down" about all this, but you did ask!' (reply 28) '... if we are able to negotiate a better contract, GPs may feel more honest about training others to join them' (reply 56), 'the morale in our group has been pretty low recently ... some are on the point of giving up' (reply 36).

One trainers group described 'having no energy left for training' (reply 9). Another respondent wanted 'more commitment from the government to listen and act on what GPs are telling them' (reply 25). They felt that being listened to would make them feel they could exert some influence on the development of training and that this would then make them feel more energetic where training was concerned.

The sense of helplessness, of feeling out of control, all the distinguishing features of burn-out were identified in some of the respondents and it appears to be connected with a perceived lack of time for anything, including teaching. A recent *British Medical Journal* showed a photograph of a frowning Asian male on its front cover with the title *Unhappy Doctors*. It contained three articles summarising doctors' views from workshops in Britain and in America.[2] Some of this unhappiness is not confined to the medical profession and has been discussed in the recent Reith Lectures which describe the erosion of public faith in professions and the breakdown of trust.[3] There is a need for an extended social study of general practice that gives a context to the problems surrounding GP morale. *Policy and Place – general medical practice in the UK* is one of the few books available that tries to do this.[4]

Remuneration

Remuneration was felt to be inadequate for the amount of time respondents felt had to be spent with the registrar. It was also felt to be inadequate compared with health authority and PCG payments for advisory or other services. Training regulations require GP trainers to spend one session a week on formal protected teaching time and one session to cover informal teaching. For this they are paid around £6000. The average sessional payment for a GP seeing patients is approximately £8000 which means teaching practices subsidise training. Typical quotes were: 'Dare I say it? More money ...' (reply 30), 'there is not enough financial resource to spend [so much] on locums to free up time to become a trainer' (reply 55).

The General Practitioners' Committee (GPC) surveyed GP trainers in 2001. Ninety-seven per cent of respondents considered that 'the training role has increased in intensity' as well as being more time consuming. The report stated that the trainer's grant 'is no longer an adequate reflection of the workload and teaching commitment involved in being a trainer, which means that currently individuals and practices are subsidising the training process ...' Only 8% of the respondents felt that the current level of grant provided adequate remuneration. The report concluded that

> ... The BMA suggest that a substantial increase in the trainer's grant would encourage GPs to become involved in training, either for the first time or by returning to it and would thus help to prevent an additional

shortfall in the number of trainers, which would undermine the possibility of meeting even the government's targets for increasing GP numbers.

Surprisingly, remuneration was the least often mentioned barrier to training in my enquiry findings. This may have been because those preparing to train are not yet in a position to gauge the amount of time and effort required to train. Alternatively, they may not have wanted to appear avaricious . . . .

Preparation to become a trainer

Many respondents stated that while 'I would also value further training/qualifications in teaching' (reply 12), there were 'too many hoops to jump through' (reply 8) to become a trainer. Preparation for training is seen as daunting.

Some criticised the inadequate notice given by the adverts and commented on the lack of information about course content. They stated it was also difficult to discover what courses might be available in the future. 'More notice is required of the courses. Previously there has been only several weeks' notice yet in a five-doctor practice our holidays have to be allocated months in advance. I have been unable to attend at least two previous courses due to lack of adequate warning.' (reply 61) 'Perhaps the dates should be available 6–9 months in advance?' (reply 19) 'Locally, our deanery does not have any information on courses that may be planned. I have been telephoning the department since February, but no one is sure when the next course might be!' (reply 22)

While doctors who had attended courses to become a trainer in SE London evaluated them extremely positively, participants perceived the time available for this activity as inadequate. Many routes to becoming trainers used in other parts of the country are not so time consuming.[5] However, the quality of the training offered needs to be of an adequate standard and this implies a major time commitment. The London Deanery now has a university accredited *Teaching the Teachers* course which, although it too appears daunting, hopefully balances the need for well prepared teachers against the pressure to produce the numbers required. There was a plethora of different courses and routes to becoming a trainer which combined with administrative difficulties during the amalgamation of four Thames deaneries led to confusion. This contributed to some potential trainers not making a commitment to train.

'There is also a feeling of things changing so quickly the goal posts are shifting and it is not exactly clear what is expected of us to become trainers.' (reply 40) 'I think for many it feels like there are lots of hurdles to get through and there is too much else going on.' (reply 4) 'I have done few modules of the trainers programme, I would like to know whether I can continue to complete the remaining modules.' (reply 27) '. . . only 3 years as a principal plus one as vocationally trained associate (VTA) so far due to working overseas. When should I start to put things in motion and what do I need to do?' (reply 32)

Respondents asked for more information about how to undertake part-time training and several new principals wanted to know when they could apply to become trainers. '. . . is part-time/job-share of training possible especially given the multiple roles of GPs and more who are working part-time (to keep their sanity!)?' (reply 59) 'I would also like to know about part-time trainers – is there facility to do this?' (reply 44)

Several respondents said their main block was that they had not passed the MRCGP examination. Its relevance was questioned: 'I do not want to spend time learning about exam structure (which I think is over-complex) rather than teaching about how to look after patients' (reply 6) and 'at this stage of my career, I am more interested in doing an MSc' (reply 62). Alternative suggestions were offered: 'I should prefer some kind of audit of my existing practice to see that I was fitted for the job of training others' (reply 17).

Infrastructure

Lack of suitable premises to accommodate a registrar was seen as a problem: 'we do not have adequate premises' (reply 26), 'because we are short of space we could only have one registrar at any one time' (reply 34). 'Physical space – two trainees: one room' (reply 58). Premises in London have improved substantially over the last 10 years, largely due to the London Implementation Zone initiatives. However, investment in teaching facilities within practices has not been made. The Department of Health has recently invested a considerable amount of money aimed at increasing space for registrars to work in. This funding can only be accessed if the practice subsequently trains, but it certainly appears to be helping to increase trainer numbers. However a lack of clarity of how it fits in with other arrangements has deflected some practices from applying for this grant. Respondents also stated they needed help with getting the practice ready for training. Note summarisation (80% have to be summarised in order to meet training criteria) was seen as a major obstacle '. . . summarising notes is a big one' (reply 51). Some PCTs across the country are trying to computerise note summarising centrally. The Department of Health has provided 'non-premises funding' to pay for this as well as help with library and video equipment if the practice either becomes a training practice or increases its capacity to train.

The philosophy/bureaucracy of training

One of the trainers groups felt that the recent changes affecting the selection of registrars had caused a great deal of confusion and lack of ownership of the process, even to the extent that it was felt that they were rather lucky to have a registrar.

The transfer of responsibility to the deanery has sent out a message, for the time being at least, that you are really rather lucky to have any registrar. It has not felt as though we are being courted, quite the opposite – it has felt as though we have had to be quite assertive to find a registrar. (reply 35)

Several commented about the 'changed ethos' of training making it much less attractive educationally, the 'year in practice now being too short' (reply 24) and 'summative assessment making registrars too task-focused' (reply 23). Several respondents expressed concern that the general practice component '. . . felt to be too crowded' and was '. . . too exam-orientated' (replies 37, 3, 71, and 21).

Respondents also criticised the trainer selection and reselection process as being too onerous and too summative.

It's the whole area of trainer reselection that seems to be preoccupying trainers. Reselection feels to be a huge obstacle. Selection by peer group review or practice visit is perceived as onerous. I wonder if it would be possible for these processes to be more formative and less summative. Also, we need help to make them simple – they seem to generate neuroticism in obsessive trainers!! (and I don't think I am just talking about myself here!!!). (reply 67)

The problems identified were discussed at London Deanery team meetings and influenced policy formation. For example, the deanery decided that non-principal experience should contribute to the qualifying experience necessary for doctors to become trainers. As a result of concern about lack of information on courses, the administrative staff now plan and advertise courses earlier. Personal contact though follow-up of concerns made the London Deanery appear less impersonal and helped establish good-will towards the Deanery. When the government announced its funding of non-premises and premises funding to encourage training practices, the survey provided names of people who had already enquired about this kind of help.

Little research appears to have been carried out on what motivates GPs to become trainers. The findings of this enquiry agree with published research and indicate what the barriers to becoming a trainer might be. The only relevant citation concerning GP teaching in the community showed that 86% of GPs have some sort of teaching experience in their current practice and a large number of medical and non-medical subjects are already being taught.[6] There was a high level of interest in UG teaching and, consequently, demand for a variety of support measures from medical schools. These included adequate financial reward, teacher training and protected time. They concluded that these issues need to be addressed '. . . if large scale changes in undergraduate teaching are to be achieved'. These findings mirror those of this enquiry.

As employees become more discerning about what they choose to use their indispensable skills for, they are asking not just 'what for?' but also 'who for?'[7]

They observe that '... the basis upon which an organisation acts, adapts and implements changes is coming to interact more and more closely with personal values'.[7] While being responsible for managing training, maintaining standards and remunerating trainers, deaneries need to understand and support the personal issues and concerns of potential trainers that this enquiry has highlighted.

The morale of trainers is important because they are the 'ambassadors' of training for general practice. A recent King's Fund survey indicated that although the personal fulfilment from training, especially in a one to one relationship, was greatly valued, there was increasing pressure by other members of the practice to question whether it was appropriate when it took the doctor away from the practice's main function, that of seeing patients.[8] Increasing time taken on training coupled with the relatively poor remuneration and lack of support from other practice members, all echoed the findings of this enquiry and the GMC survey.

The motivation to become a trainer is the key to encouraging the taking up of this role. The professionalisation of the role of the teacher in general practice began in 1977 and has been described by Stevens.[9] In 1980, a survey conducted in Cambridgeshire Health Authority found that undergraduate GP teachers graduated more recently, subscribed to more journals and were more likely to use medical libraries. Also, single-handed and two-person practices belonged to a subgroup of non-teachers suggesting that it was difficult to become a trainer in a smaller practice.[10] This is relevant as London has a large proportion of single-handed and two-partner practices. This study also poses the question whether students stimulate trainers to read or whether this is a characteristic of an enquiring, self-motivated group.

Recent attention to the positive aspects of PPD provided by a teaching role may be another way of encouraging GPs to become teachers. A profile of Peter Toon, a medical educationalist, provides an attractive picture of teaching enriching all areas of professional life. 'My type of career is however, fun and never boring'.[11] In the same supplement another article starts with 'you are in your mid-thirties, you qualified as a doctor ten years ago, and although you are still enjoying medical practice, you are starting to think about introducing more variety to your every day work to lighten the daily grind. Why not consider medical education?' and continues by describing becoming a trainer amongst other teaching roles.[12]

An article entitled 'why do trainers train?' described in-depth interviews with five trainers in order to establish their reason for wanting to train.[13] Although the survey was small it highlighted four areas of training which these trainers found rewarding: trainer-centred factors, registrar-centred factors, practice-centred factors and professionally-centred factors. The survey concentrates more on the rewards gained once training is undertaken rather than the barriers to be overcome to start training. However, understanding the personal satisfaction to be gained from being a trainer might be used to motivate doctors to train.

Child described questions that might be asked to help understand why someone is motivated to do something. What is the internal need that this action is trying to satisfy? What result is this action trying to achieve? With what degree of energy or enthusiasm is this action being undertaken?[14] Working with potential trainers individually might allow sensitive exploration of motives to enhance an individual's commitment to training.

Maslow's hierarchy of needs explains why GPs are unable to satisfy '... higher needs such as self-expression and creativity', when more basic needs of being in control are not there.[15] McCleland and colleagues introduced the concept of achievement motivation which correlates with some identified GP needs, to continue to achieve in what can be seen as a very flat career path (potentially years with the same title and status).[16]

Ausubel had already described at least three components of achievement motivation in: 'cognitive drive' where the individual attempts to satisfy the need to know and understand, 'self enhancement' representing a desire for

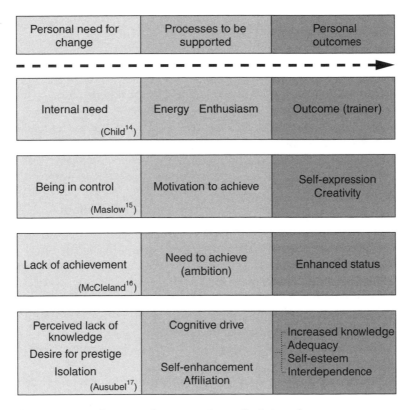

Figure 6.2   Motivating doctors to become trainers: the internal process.

increased prestige and status leading to feelings of adequacy and self-esteem, 'affiliation' a broad need for relationships with and therefore dependence on other people.[17] Affiliation could be emphasised when recruiting trainers, as the sense of belonging to a group with a similar task is greatly valued by trainers from their membership of 'workshops'. These are small groups which meet, usually monthly, to support each other in their role as trainers and to increase their skills. When a trainer's wife died recently, the trainer wrote that the fellowship he felt at being part of a workshop fraternity was more important to him than he would ever have believed.

Figure 6.2 shows how these different theories might be used to facilitate doctors becoming trainers and may explain why, in spite of all the barriers, some doctors do take up this role.

Recommendations

Recommendations may be considered under each of the six categories of barriers to becoming a trainer that the enquiry identified.

Lack of time

Free up doctors' time to teach and time to prepare for teaching by:

- release of doctor by vocationally trained associate-type schemes[18] and GP assistant/research associate schemes[19]
- increasing supply of locums by supporting PCT-based locum banks that provide peer support and protected education time for locums e.g. buddy scheme, mentoring scheme
- reducing practice list size in training practices without affecting remuneration.

Low morale of GPs

- build on success of local peer support groups and mentoring schemes
- increase protected learning time schemes
- promote the 'life enhancing' aspects of training by recruiting existing trainers to describe the role
- develop teaching practices in collaboration with PCTs, workforce confederation and the deanery
- enhance the status of trainers and teaching practices.

Remuneration

- negotiations by GMC to increase remuneration for trainers
- perhaps a bounty for inner-city trainers.

Preparation

- PCT, confederation and deanery support for obtaining membership of the RCGP (MRCGP) via the 'membership by assessment of performance' route (a formative process that raises the standard of the whole practice)
- local support groups (LSGs) for aiding the development of those interested in education (Bromley model)
- define a clearer, more coherent pathway to becoming a trainer
- integrate UG and PG qualifications to produce a career ladder from UG teaching to PG teaching
- integrate/overlap undergraduate and postgraduate educational qualifications
- training to be undertaken by part-time and job-sharing doctors
- introduce a 'buddy system' for potential trainers.

Infrastructure of training

- collaboration between PCT, confederation and deanery to distribute funding for premises development and non-premises support to practices preparing to become training practices
- develop the concept of 'accredited teaching practices' with PCTs, confederation and deanery to support the teaching of all members of the primary care team
- 'road shows' to visit PCTs to describe the rewards of the role, the route to becoming a trainer and the support available.

Philosophy/bureaucracy of training

- make the training process more supportive and formative rather than summative
- lobby the GMC and RCGP to simplify the vocational training process to become a GP. (Summative assessment is felt to be too onerous when combined with the MRCGP in registrar year.)
- reduce bureaucracy of becoming and remaining a trainer.

Taking things further

The participants in the UKCEA workshop were invited to brainstorm how training capacity might be increased and the following additional ideas emerged:

- ask PCTs 'who are your best practices that are not already training?'
- send questionnaires to GPs 'what stops you becoming trainers?' in a similar way to that described above
- use Department of Health premises and non-premises funding effectively
- encourage WDCs to invest in practices as learning organisations for both medical and non-medical clinical placements
- develop the concept of an 'associate trainer', that is someone preparing to become a trainer (as has already been piloted in some deaneries)
- devolve the summarising of notes centrally to the PCT (as already carried out in one PCT)
- take care when attaching PRHOs to practices as damage can easily be done to individuals and organisational relationships
- rename SHO posts for general practice training
- PCTs to fund relevant GP SHO posts e.g. in palliative care, drug addiction, refuges etc. (as already developed in some areas)
- PCTs and deaneries collaborate to fund attachments to relevant GP training in the registrar year
- hold a separate GP recruitment fair annually.

Conclusion

The challenge to increase the number of GPs raises complex issues that go beyond simply increasing training capacity, the strategy currently being pursued by government and deaneries. For example, when 50% of graduates will become GPs why are hospitals so reluctant to provide appropriate SHO posts? Why do the new SHO structures proposed pay scant regard to describing how the new arrangements will improve GP training? How will the new Postgraduate Medical Education and Training Board (PMETB) monitor the quality and appropriateness of GP training? Will a new GP contract raise the morale of GPs and also make general practice a more attractive career option? Deaneries need courage and flexibility to meet the challenges ahead as well as resources in terms of money and time.

With the proposed reorganisation of the SHO years there are many imponderables.[20] Any change will mean a radical shake-up of the hospital experience for those wishing to become GPs. It will also mean that in the foundation years every graduate may be offered the opportunity to spend time in general practice, bringing attendant pressure on trainers and training practices.

For education to be relevant for general practice there needs to be a great deal of preparation. Elsewhere in this book Souster and Savage describe (Chapter 3) essential components for successful SHO education for general practice. Learning outcomes will need to be clear and educational supervision, so vital to success, will need to be supported both with time and expertise.

As the *European Working Time Directive* and other European Union (EU) edicts impinge on SHO work patterns the relevance of hospital SHO-based education for general practice may be brought into question. Successful integration of community-based training within hospital SHO posts has provided relevant training that has proved popular. At present, funding training in community trusts is extremely difficult.

Course organisers will need to become increasingly expert at brokering appropriate placements in higher professional education where a programme director has been appointed. This may need to be a new title for course organisers to reflect much more what they will need to do.

From the experience of SLOVTS we have learnt that in order to develop innovative SHO training the relationship between consultant and course organiser is key. There is no guarantee with the new arrangements envisaged that consultants will be any more willing to provide posts for those seeking a career in general practice (although this reluctance may be a teaching hospital phenomenon).

The preoccupation with creating new posts may overlook the careful planning and imaginative use of resources needed for optimal development of SHO education. The experience of converting trust posts to vocational training emphasises the conflict between service and education. Hospitals reliant on trust-funded SHOs did not find it easy to support the educational component needed to make the posts beneficial to the learner.

The rhetoric envisages exciting possibilities and certainly there is great opportunity for collaborative education development between the hospital and primary care. The proposals also acknowledge the need to integrate undergraduate training with the first years of postgraduate training. The government has seen fit to measure medical school performance using research criteria. Teachers who do little or no research are being 'let go', teaching staff are being reduced by up to a third while student admission rates are being increased and more multidisciplinary teaching is being undertaken. There is no direct correlation between a good researcher and a good teacher. It is not known how these changes will alter the quality of graduates from our medical schools in the future. Against this background, general practice needs to be very clear about what training and skills are needed for the future GP.

'Numbers' is the current political imperative and it is one that service GPs have great sympathy for when trying to attract new partners, assistants or locums to see the patients who do not stop coming just because there are not enough primary care team members to see them. So the numbers are vital but the standard of care given to patients must be remembered also. Curricula and assessment seek external demonstrable standards but doctors also need to develop self-direction and internal motivations to develop as autonomous professionals. The balance between service and education has never seemed so important but so fragile.

References

1   Harnady W and Wickson J (1981) Religion at our age, an interview with William Harnady, PhD. *Modern Maturity.* **24**: 27.

2   Edwards N, Cornachie MJ and Silversin J (2002) Unhappy doctors: what are the causes and what can be done? *BMJ.* **324**: 835.

3   O'Neill O (2002) Reith Lectures. BBC Radio 4. (www.bbc.co.uk/radio4/reith2002/)

4   Moon G and North N (2000) *Policy and Place – general medical practice in the UK.* McMillan Press Ltd, London.

5   Freeman R, Smith F and Hornung R (2002) Courses for new GP trainers: a literature review and survey for the UK CRA. *Educ Prim Care.* **13**: 1–12.

6   Gray J and Fine B (1997) A study of teaching experience and interest in undergraduate teaching in the future. *Br J Gen Pract.* **47**: 623–6.

7   Maybee GBC (1993) Facilitating radical change. In: C Maybee and B Mayon-White (eds) *Managing Change.* Paul Chapman Publishing Ltd, London.

8   Osborne K and Green J (2001) *Increasing the Capacity for GP Registrar Training in London.* Health Services Research Unit, London School of Hygiene and Tropical Medicine, London.

9   Stevens G (1977) On becoming a teacher of family medicine. *J Fam Pract.* **4**: 325–7.

10 Hay J, Acheson RM, Reiss BB and Evans CE (1980) Teachers in general practice: a comparative study. *Med Educ.* **14**: 277–84.

11 Toon P (2002) *Profile BMJ Career Focus.* **324**: 570.

12 Chambers R, Mohana K and Field S (2002) A career in medical education – looking to broaden your horizons while sharpening your brain? *BMJ Career Focus.* **324**: 565.

13 Spencer Jones R (1997) Why do trainers train? *Educ Gen Pract.* **8**: 31–9.

14 Child E (1993) *Human Motivation in Psychology and the Teacher.* p. 35–71, Castle, London.

15 Maslow AH (1970) *Motivation and Personality.* Harper and Rowe, New York.

16 McCleland DC, Atkinson JW, Clark RA and Lovell EJ (1976) *The Achievement Motive.* Irving Publishers, New York.

17 Ausubel DP and Robinson FG (1969) *School Learning.* Holt, Reinhart and Winston, New York.

18 Salmon E and Savage R (1997) The vocationally trained associate (VTA) scheme: outcomes after the first 2 years – (i) the VTAs. *Educ Gen Pract.* **8**: 191–8.

19 Bellman L and Morley V (2001) GPs in transition: the GP assistant/research associate scheme. Kings College/Bayswater Institute joint publication, London.

20 Donaldson Sir L (2002) *Unfinished Business – proposals for reform of the Senior House Officer grade.* (www.doh.gov.uk/shoconsult/)

Further reading

- Department of Health. *The NHS Plan.* (www.nhs.uk/nationalplan/contents.htm)

- Department of Health, NHS workforce statistics. (www.doh.gov.uk/nhs.workforce.htm)

- Marinker M (ed.) (1994) *Controversies in Health Care Policies. Challenges to practice.* BMJ Publishing Group, London.

- Maybee C and Mayon-White B (eds) (1993) *Managing Change.* Paul Chapman Publishing Ltd, London.

- Mertens DM (1998) *Research Methods in Education and Psychology: integrating diversity with quantitative and qualitative approaches.* Sage Publications, Thousand Oaks, California.

Thanks are extended to the workshop participants.

CHAPTER 7

Senior registrars in general practice in Kent, Surrey and Sussex

Kevin Hurrell

Introduction

Kent, Surrey and Sussex (KSS) Deanery started its senior GP registrar scheme in August 2001, initially as a pilot programme, to support the recruitment and retention of GP principals in their area. The scheme offers registrars who have completed summative assessment a further six months' training at senior registrar level. Senior GP registrars (SGPRs) are expected to spend 40% of their time exploring areas outside their training practice but within the wider terrain of the NHS. This may constitute further clinical experience within secondary care, perhaps with a view to later specialisation, or within public health or perhaps attached to their local primary care organisations (PCOs).

This chapter arises from a workshop given at the 2002 UKCEA conference. The workshop was designed to explore the thinking and ideology behind the scheme and outline the process of the scheme up to the present time. It highlighted the views of those presently participating in the scheme, that is SGPRs, trainers and myself as course organiser. It explored the experiences and the views of those involved in similar schemes elsewhere in the country. The workshop also looked to the future, explored possible further developments and looked to some of the potential problems and attempted to find some solutions.

The KSS senior GP registrar scheme

The scheme began in August 2001 with a view to tackling problems of recruitment and retention of GPs across Kent, Surrey and Sussex. It was designed to offer support to registrars as they 'bridged the gap between supervised and independent working, and to give them the opportunity to specialise'. It was designed to encourage the pursuit of academic qualifications and give these high flyers enhanced status.

There are other spin-offs too, in particular those around the areas of recruitment and retention. Up to 40% of new GPs have left practice within three years, and the BMA estimates there were only an additional 18 full-time equivalent GPs across the whole country recruited last year. The KSS Deanery recognises that future GPs will expect flexible working practices and will pursue something of a 'portfolio career'. There are specific areas within Kent, Surrey and Sussex with even greater problems of recruitment and these problems are increased by high levels of retirement. It is hoped that the SGPR scheme will encourage doctors to look more favourably upon these areas, as they remain an additional six months in their locality.

Structure and process

Senior registrars have a further six months with a training practice. This may be their own, but they are encouraged to look elsewhere in order to gain the widest possible exposure to general practice. Up to 40% of the week however is spent exploring areas outside general practice, for instance in another clinical speciality, an area of research or through involvement with another healthcare organisation. SGPRs attend a regular day release programme and are expected to report back upon the progress of their personal development plan (PDP) throughout their six months, and to submit a written report at the end of their term.

The day release is co-ordinated by a course organiser who promotes the scheme, supports, advises and ultimately appoints applicants. The course organiser liaises regularly with trainers, other course organisers and other agencies and has links throughout the deanery team. New and emergent relationships with others involved in education have also been formed, such as those with the HPE programme directors.

The day release programme belongs to the senior registrars and reflects their status. It encourages group identity and support and demands their own contribution. It is varied in content and format and is fun!

Current situation and the future

Eighteen senior registrars have been appointed so far and four of them have actually completed their six months. There is an increased awareness of the scheme and many more applications are in the pipeline. Feedback so far has been very positive and the aims of the scheme do seem to be realised. All current senior registrars are planning to take MRCGP and some are acquiring specialist qualifications as well.

We can build upon the present sound structure and further refine the scheme while celebrating its success to date. The scheme needs to collaborate with the educational programme being organised by the KSS Deanery for new doctors in general practice and it is hoped that all senior registrars will move on and join the HPE scheme organised within the KSS area. The senior registrar scheme should just be one link in a chain of educational opportunity within the deanery 'family' which supports doctors throughout the whole of their career.

Discussion

Sharing the KSS experience with colleagues operating similar schemes around the country has highlighted a number of issues. Positive and negative points emerge as well as a number of interesting and less easily resolved questions.

Undoubtedly, such a scheme permits an opportunity for GP registrars to plug gaps in their knowledge or experience. This further period of security allows the registrar time to take stock, mature as an individual and reflect on their personal development. There is the chance to explore new relationships and undergo experiences that act to increase status and confidence. The result is a powerful catalyst for change.

However, such a scheme is expensive and we must consider whether it attracts added value. There is delay in getting registrars off the starting blocks and into the professional workplace, and the pool of young GP locums may be consequently depleted. The secure nature of the scheme could also conceivably delay the necessary maturation of an individual doctor by the very fact it is so protected. Concerns have also been raised about the exploitation of the scheme to the advantage of applicants contemplating a period of maternity leave.

Various issues around selection emerge. Some deaneries clearly try to attract high flyers. Others accept applications at random to ensure a mixed cross section. There are merits in both approaches but deaneries perhaps need to be clear whether they are responding to need and distributive justice across geographical areas, or simply concerned with promoting excellence.

The role of the training practice is also interesting. Should non-trainers be involved with the supervision of senior registrars? If not, why not, since these doctors have already satisfied the requirements of summative assessment and are – in theory at least – fit for independent practice. And what about the trainer's grant? Currently it is only possible to pay one trainer's grant to an individual trainer regardless of the number or type of GP registrars they take, but this is an ideal opportunity for a trainer to take on overlapping registrars, thus creating valuable increased training capacity. For the present time, at least, it appears that we are limited in flexibility by regulation, and senior registrars and the financial arrangements concerning them are treated in the same way as other vocational trainees.

With so many schemes emerging over the country, some evaluation will be necessary. But there are difficulties in doing so. How do you compare with the norm when the norm is not monitored? If you pick out the high flyers then aren't they likely to succeed anyway? It is relatively easy to show what proportion of senior registrars remain in general practice in the months and years following their involvement with the scheme. Although such data might be useful, its statistical significance would be hard to prove. There is clearly a need to share best practice and the results of evaluation across the UK.

In the KSS Deanery we recognise the need to link senior registrar training to a more wide-reaching higher professional education programme. From discussion at the 2002 UKCEA conference, other deaneries around the country appear to concur. If this is to be the case, then senior registrars may represent an interim arrangement on the way to providing a more seamless pathway of professional development. So catch them while you can!

Based on a workshop given at the 2002 UKCEA conference. With thanks to the participants Drs Jas Bilkhu, Mike Grenville, N Jackson, Malcolm Lewis, B Lewis, Anthea Lints, Aly Rashid and Rebecca Viney.

CHAPTER 8

Flexible training for general practice

Anne Hastie

Flexible training often has a low priority in postgraduate departments of general practice, possibly because of the relatively small numbers involved. Doctors of both sexes are eligible for flexible training if they have well founded reasons, such as young children or disability. The number of doctors applying for flexible training is increasing each year as more women qualify and many want to work part-time.[1] They must be of equivalent ability to those doing full-time posts and should be interviewed with reference to equal opportunities.

The London Deanery is large and has two Associate Deans (ADs) of Postgraduate Medicine working exclusively with hospital flexible training, including SHO posts. They work closely with the Deputy Dean of Postgraduate General Practice who has responsibility for flexible GP vocational training. Many other deaneries do not appear to have lead ADs but this may reflect their smaller number of flexible trainees.

The majority of flexible trainees are supernumerary, although there are a few substantive flexible training posts. Doctors apply to the deanery for flexible training funding and if approved can use the funding to organise an educationally approved post. The process for educational approval is the same as full-time SHO posts and requires help from the DPGPE or nominated deputy. For general practice training the SHO post must be at least 60% of the time and duties of full-time SHOs in similar employment. There must be at least one week of whole-time employment relating to the prescribed period of hospital training.[2]

The deaneries control the funds for flexible training SHO posts, although the trusts have to pay for the out of hours work. Those working less than 40 hours per week are placed in one of three flexible bands:[3]

- FC – working only between 8 am and 7 pm. This is paid strictly pro-rata and paid in full from the deanery flexible training budget

- FB – full basic salary plus a multiplier of 0.05
- FA – full basic salary plus a multiplier of 0.25.

For band FB and FC the deanery pay the pro-rata salary and the trust has to fund the remainder of the basic salary plus the multiplier. This is a great disincentive for trusts to employ flexible trainees and has led to problems throughout the deaneries. Temporary financial help from the Department of Health came into place in August 2002 to enable deaneries to fund up to 100% of the basic salary in compliant posts.

Problems can arise when doctors appointed to a VTS ask to change to flexible training. These are usually handled on an individual basis with the help of the course organisers, but can be time consuming and complex. The London Deanery has been trying to organise some flexible training VTSs, but so far has only managed one formal scheme based at St George's with accident and emergency, care of the elderly and a GP registrar post. Trusts are reluctant to co-operate because of the length of time it takes a flexible trainee to complete the rotation and the possibility of doctors leaving during the scheme.

Organising flexible training as a GP registrar is less difficult as the deanery controls the payments in full. Anecdotally those trainers who have employed a part-time GP registrar have generally felt positive about the experience. Again the flexible trainee must work at least 60% of the equivalent full-time post, with at least one week of whole-time employment.[2]

Bullying and disability may be a problem for some flexible trainees. Many deaneries, including the London Deanery, have a written bullying protocol[4] and deaneries could consider sharing each other's guidelines. The *Disability Discrimination Act* is important and deaneries can apply for a Disability Friendly Badge through their local Disability Office. Funding can be obtained from the Department of Employment through the Disability Employment Adviser towards aids for disabled employees.

Flexible trainees (as well as full-time trainees) who have health problems need the support of an occupational health service. It is important that those supporting the trainee liaise with each other and there are examples where this has not happened. Equal opportunities should be taken into account when interviewing and appointing doctors with disability. When problems arise with bullying or discrimination the BMA may become involved, especially if the trainee seeks their help. It is much better if deaneries have systems in place, which avoid these problems.

Flexible training is an increasingly important part of the work performed by deaneries and, with the feminisation of the medical workforce, is set to become more prominent still. Experience in London suggests that the organisation of the current complex arrangements works more efficiently if a named person takes a lead responsibility and acquires an extensive knowledge of the subject.

References

1 Allen I (1994) *Doctors and their Careers: a new generation*. Policy Studies Institute, London.

2 Joint Committee on Postgraduate Training for General Practice (JCPTGP) (1998) *Guidelines on Flexible (Part Time) Training for General Practice*. JCPTGP, London.

3 Department of Health (2000) *Modernising Pay and Contracts for Hospital Doctors and Dentists in Training*. DoH, London.

4 London Postgraduate Medical and Dental Education (2000) *Dignity at Work*. LPMDE, London.

Based on an open space workshop at the 2002 UKCEA conference.

CHAPTER 9

Practicalities in delivering higher professional education in the London Deanery

Tareq Abouharb

A GP who has only recently completed vocational training and is entering practice has many challenges to overcome. The pressures engendered by this period of transition have led to the development of a formalised period of extended support: higher professional education (HPE). The need for HPE is recurrently documented, with key papers demonstrating both the sudden loss of educational support post-vocational training, and the range of need required.[1–5]

The London Deanery HPE programme came on-stream in October 2001 in the face of an additional significant challenge. The deanery had just formed as a coalescence of the four preceding Thames Postgraduate GP Departments, and now encompassed what seemed like a vast range in diversity of patient- and doctor-need. This chapter describes how HPE has been implemented in London, the problems that have arisen and possible future developments.

The London HPE team

A team of HPE programme directors, two for each of the London Deanery's five workforce sectors, were appointed in 2001. In each sector, one programme director is nominally dedicated to new non-principals, the other to new principals. A task-orientated AD supports the programme directors, with a Deputy Dean overseeing the project. A full-time dedicated administrative manager takes care of paper flow and application queries.

The team undertook a series of induction workshops focusing on evolving agreed team strategy, operational issues, developing a deeper understanding of reflective learning and PDPs. The programme directors are establishing links with course organisers and GP tutors in their sector, and are planning to participate in a sector-wide group forum of educationalists.

The educational challenge

Making the process and content of HPE relevant is key to connecting with and addressing the needs of its end users. It is interesting how the national experience of HPE curriculum content has been broadly similar. The mode of delivery, and whether it is accredited for use towards higher degrees, have been the main differences.[5,6]

The London Deanery HPE format takes its basis from the original recommendations made in Professor Janet Grant's report,[4] suggesting the need for a wide range of educational opportunities, that can be accessed in a variety of ways over a period of years. We are planning for an individual to be supported for two years, at a minimum of 10 days per year.

The HPE team has developed a user pack and an end of vocational training assessment tool to evaluate learning needs on entry to the HPE scheme. The pack and assessment tool are available at (www.londondeanery.ac.uk/gp). Identified needs are carried forward into a PDP, in keeping with the aims outlined by the Chief Medical Officer in 1998.[7] The aim of HPE is to encourage skills acquisition that will prove beneficial for ongoing professional development of the individual in their primary healthcare team, thus taking into account the diversity of challenge they may encounter working in their locality.[8] This linking of personal development to practice development serves to better integrate and support a new GP with the reality of their workplace. In addition, it fosters mutual respect between the new GP and primary care team as the practice benefits from the added value that the new GP's learning brings to the organisation.

The PDP of each new GP is actioned in a way to fit with their commitments and opportunities. The use of secondments, self-directed learning groups and learning in individual practices is positively encouraged. The drive throughout is to move from the structure of vocational training to a reflective self-directed learning within a supportive peer group.

The curriculum

The London Deanery HPE team has developed a basic list of suggested topics (*see* Box) with which to cross reference when establishing the learner's needs. Rather than providing a fixed curriculum, the topics form a starting point from which individuals can evolve their PDPs having undertaken their learning needs assessment. The programme directors in each London sector then run half-day release workshops on topics of shared need, but individuals may wish to address their other learning objectives in a variety of self-directed modalities, as detailed previously. The aim is to produce a personalised curriculum relevant to the individual, with the purpose of reinforcing the broad base of the generalist, whilst leaving scope to develop areas of primary care specialism.

Curriculum topics in HPE

Performance
- Appraisal and personal development planning
- Preparing for revalidation
- Practice professional development plans
- Clinical governance/health improvement programme (HImP)/National Service Framework (NSF)

Medicine and the law
- Partnership agreements/joining a practice
- Medico-legal dilemmas
- Ethical dilemmas
- Contractual agreements in the modern NHS (GMS/PMS etc.)

Practice management and finance
- Recruitment and employment law
- Personal finance
- Practice finance/accounts and claims

Skills
- IT/presentation skills
- Consultation skills/communication skills
- Creative problem solving
- Negotiation skills and assertiveness training
- Time and stress management
- Audit and research
- Report writing
- Secondary care provision in primary care
- Information gathering/critical reading skills
- Practising evidence-based medicine

Self-directed personal development and reflective learning
- Career planning
- Mentoring
- Optimising self-directed learning/self-directed learning groups
- Higher degrees/support for education

Overcoming barriers to HPE uptake

The profile of doctors taking up general practice in the UK has changed dramatically over the past two decades. There has been a steady fall in the proportion of male GPs, and the number of all GPs becoming principals has halved.[9] In London, female GPs form 60% of entrants and are keener to work part-time, with only 18% choosing to be principals in the first instance. In addition, new GPs are less likely to remain in the area within which they completed their training.[10] The effect of this demographic change is that of a need to dramatically increase the number of new GPs trained, with 150 registrars required for each 100 GPs retiring.[11] There is also an implicit need to try and retain GPs in the area within which they are training, and provide incentives for recruitment wherever possible.

It becomes self-evident then that newer GPs are seeking a lifestyle with greater flexibility, less early commitment to partnership, and experimenting as non-principals in a variety of geographical locations. Delivering HPE thus needs to take these factors into account, and facilitate support of learning in protected time when the individual would have otherwise been committed to service provision. Maintaining service provision where there are shortages in locum colleagues to cover causes a significant problem for new GPs attempting to

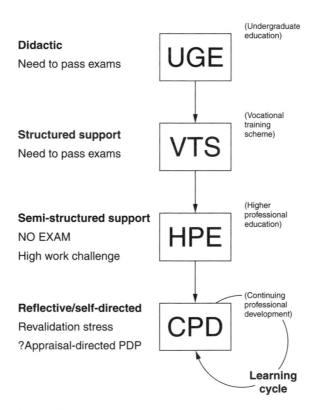

Figure 9.1 Learning continuum.

engage in HPE. This is compounded by present locum replacement expenses (£250 per day) being too low for the reality of London costs. Some new GPs report that senior partners are reluctant to allow them HPE time out in addition to any pre-existing study leave arrangements, such that it has become vital for new GPs to negotiate HPE time into their contract or partnership agreement from the outset.

A further complication reducing uptake is failure to make contact with new GP non-principals that have entered the London area after completing vocational training and possibly registered on supplementary lists elsewhere, that we cannot identify. The quality of the data recorded on supplementary lists is still variable, and with HPE often coinciding with a time when GPs move home and across health authority or PCT boundaries, databases rapidly become outdated.

As was highlighted at the Third Cambridge Conference on Higher Professional Education in March 2002, the national picture was for lower than expected uptake of HPE. Figures of 25–50% uptake were quoted, with as yet no definite cause established for such a low figure. Uptake in London has been difficult to quote in percentage terms as the exact total eligible is yet to be accurately established due to incomplete supplementary list data, but our present working estimate of 410, with uptake thus far of 96, yields an approximate 24%.

There is a change in emphasis in the educational continuum (Figure 9.1) at the HPE stage; a new GP is for the first time not having to work for an exam and there may be an element of 'demob-happy' rebellion. The new GP may also perceive themselves to be in survival mode and too busy to learn. Both of these factors may contribute to disengagement from education. It is certainly established that participation in learning drops off in the first year after becoming a principal, to then become much better focused in the second year.[4] The precise reasons for this remain conjecture until our first year evaluation is completed.

Future developments

The London HPE team has resolved to better connect with new GPs in five ways:

1 to set up an automated first mailing with information and pack to GP registrars nearing completion of vocational training
2 to follow up the mailing with a 'one-to-one' meeting for entry learning needs assessment where the new GP is to be given the opportunity to clarify how to get the best out of HPE
3 to simplify the application process as much as possible
4 to use web-based resources, and publicise via trainers, course organisers and tutors to raise the profile of HPE at the 'coal face'
5 to set up launch day events in each sector.

Conclusion

At the time of writing, the London Deanery HPE programme has been running for nine months. A user pack, learning needs assessment tool and outline curriculum topics have been established and a network of programme directors appointed. Early feedback on uptake has already reshaped the application process, resulting in some simplification. Uptake in London has been broadly in line with the national experience and recent discussions at the 2002 UKCEA conference have been most valuable to reflect on the barriers to HPE uptake and how best to address them. Formal evaluation of the London Deanery HPE project at the end of its first year will further inform planning.

References

1 Department of Health (1968) *Royal Commission on Medical Education*. Department of Health, London.

2 Jackson N and Reiss M (1998) *Higher Professional Education for General Practice. A report for COGPED on current work in the UK* (unpublished).

3 Royal College of General Practitioners (1998) *An Evaluation of Educational Needs and Provision for Doctors within Three Years of Completion of Vocational Training*. RCGP, London.

4 Grant J, Flood S, Mack J *et al.* (1998) *Final Report: An Evaluation of Educational Needs and Provision for Doctors within Three Years of Completion of Vocational Training for General Practice*. Joint Centre for Education in Medicine, London.

5 Smith L, Eve R and Crabtree R (2000) Higher professional education for general medical practitioners. *Br J Gen Pract*. **50**: 293–8.

6 Baron R, McKinlay D, Martin J *et al.* (2001) Higher professional education for GPs in the North West of England – feedback from the first three years. *Educ Prim Care*. **12**: 421–9.

7 Chief Medical Officer (1998) *A Review of Continuing Professional Development in General Practice*. Department of Health, London.

8 Grant J (2002) Learning needs assessment: assessing the need. *BMJ*. **324**: 156–9.

9 Lambert T, Evans J, Goldacre M *et al.* (2002) Recruitment of UK-trained doctors into general practice: findings from national cohort studies. *Br J Gen Pract*. **52**: 364–71.

10 Bowler I and Jackson N (2002) Experiences and career intentions of general practice registrars in Thames deaneries: postal survey. *BMJ*. **324**: 464–5.

11 Royal College of General Practitioners (1997) *The Primary Care Workforce. A descriptive analysis*. RCGP, London.

Based on a workshop given at the 2002 UKCEA conference. With thanks to the workshop participants, Drs Neil Jackson, Anne Hastie, Freddy Shaw, Ted Leverton, Ed Peile, John Pitts, Stewart Wilkie, Paul Bowie, Steve Hiew, Sharaf Kasimov, Nadira Nasritdinova, Dilya Sadikhodgajeva, Nargiza Saidova.

CHAPTER 10

Workforce development in general practice and primary care – past, present and future

Charles Easmon

Keynote speech delivered at the 2002 UKCEA conference

Thank you for inviting me to speak to you at the start of this conference. We have all been through a period of intense change and turbulence in the field of clinical education and development. The only thing that is certain is that there is no immediate prospect of reaching equilibrium or stasis. Change has become a way of life and we must learn to live with it, even thrive on it. Unfortunately change tends to be accompanied these days by a disparaging of history, a feeling that we have nothing to learn from the past except perhaps excuses for not being more enthusiastic about the future. The corporate memory of the system is also being lost. This is important because the continuity that you all represent is one repository of corporate memory. The past cannot tell us about the future, but learning from it can prevent us repeating the same mistakes.

   PG deaneries and WDCs will have to work ever more closely together. This will not be an easy process. To date in many parts of the country the legacy of a system of clinical professional training that almost completely separated medical from non-medical training is still with us. The PG medical education system is complex and those new to it, such as the WDCs, will naturally question the need for all this complexity. They are also organisations with a predominantly managerial culture, very different from that of the average deanery. The two cultures do not necessarily share the same points of reference. One is new, the other well established. One is used with contracts and large systems, the other with individuals and the intricacies of individual need. The meeting of the two is almost bound to be stormy. I would go so far as to say that if there is not a deal of turbulence in your early relationship with WDCs then it is probably too superficial and you are not getting to the heart of joint effective working. From the show of hands I see that only some of you have thus far had any significant contact and that so far all is generally harmonious. I suggest many of you have quite a journey ahead.

As you make it, remember that the challenge that will come to your way of doing things is healthy and natural, even where the tone may seem abrasive. You have one critical piece of common ground. Both the deanery and the WDC are advocates of the importance of workforce development to the delivery of high quality patient care. The NHS does not have a tradition of recognising the central place of workforce development, regarding it as an optional extra or arcane special interest. You both have a common interest in changing that. Keep that common interest in mind as you explore ways of working together.

I have for many years believed that if PG deaneries did not exist they would have to be invented. You will all be comfortable with that, more so perhaps than with what follows, which is 'but today what would we invent?'. What I mean by this is to open up the question of form and function. Our comfort zone is always form – structures and processes, rather than function. What should be the function of the GP side of a PG deanery in the twenty-first century? Are your skills and competencies appropriate for the needs of a service and society wanting more patient focus, involvement and convenience, more team working, greater flexibility in how the team works and who does what, and more assessment of the competence of practitioners, for supporting a clinical workforce that wants better and more flexible working conditions, continued clinical autonomy and greater involvement in service decisions? With all this change what will be the role of the doctor in the future, let alone that of the GP? The WDCs will be asking about your future purpose, about how far you see your role in developing primary care, not just general practice, and whether your deanery is fit for that purpose.

Deanery history

It is worth reviewing briefly deanery history. The creation of PG deans and regional advisers in general practice had its origins in the Christchurch Conference in the early sixties. The responsibilities on the GP side were broader, covering both the developments in vocational training and the contractual changes that led to the establishment of the Postgraduate Education Allowance (PGEA). The working paper that covered postgraduate medical education (PGME) following *Working for Patients* in 1989 set out the new arrangements for both hospital and general practice. This was followed in 1992 by the Executive Letter *EL (92) 63* which provided the financial underpinning of hospital PGME, including those SHO posts linked with vocational training, and gave the regional advisers in general practice access to infrastructure funding to help support the expanding network of trainers, course organisers and tutors and administrative support. Since then MADEL was introduced (1996). Regional advisers became directors of postgraduate GP education (DPGPEs), CRAGPIE changed to COGPED and the funding for the remainder of PG GP training moved from GMS to MADEL. The only significant change to deaneries came two years after the change to regional office structures in the south of England with the formation of a London deanery, a Kent Surrey Sussex and an Eastern Deanery and last year when the MADEL element of the MPET levy started to flow through the WDCs.

History behind workforce development confederations

What about the WDCs? Their origins can be traced back to Working Paper 10 of *Working for Patients*.[1] This covered the education and training of clinical professional staff other than doctors and dentists. It recommended moving this out of the NHS and into higher education, with the regional health authorities (RHAs) establishing contracts with higher education institutions for this training. There were then 14 RHAs. The process had no central guidelines or support so each RHA set out to do this in its own way and at its own pace. The result was a multiplicity of contract types and prices, not necessarily covering the same things. Often the NHS lacked the in-house expertise to handle the process on the basis of quality, so it was decided on price. In some areas there was competitive tendering, in others none. Some RHAs completed the process in a short time, while others took years. In 1993/4 the then NHS Management Executive set up the *Functions and Manpower Review*. This endorsed the principle of transferring the education of non-medical clinical professionals to higher education, but also stated that NHS employers were too distant from the process of staff education and should be directly involved in the contracting with higher education, which at that time was largely carried out by the RHAs not the employers. With the abolition of the RHAs and the moving of many of their functions into the NHS Executive as regional offices in 1996, together with the creation of the NMET levy which funded the contracting process, there was a need to create a system that could take on the role of the RHA. The answer was the creation of Education and Training Consortia, collaboratives of NHS employers (trusts) plus NHS commissioners (health authorities). The consortia were given the responsibility of managing the education contracts and the NMET levy, initially supervised closely by the NHS Executive through the regional offices. Although the letter setting this out *EL (95) 27*[2] stated that PG deaneries and others such as social services and the independent and voluntary sectors should be a part of the consortia, this did not happen to any great degree. Two years after their introduction consortia were allowed to manage their affairs independently of regional offices subject to proving their competence so to do.

Education consortia were fine in principle and the best of them did some excellent innovative work. However they had a number of built-in weaknesses.

- The primary aim of *EL (95) 27*[2] was to have a mechanism for the management of the NMET levy. It was long on process, but short on the vision of what such a collaborative might be. The most successful consortia tried to develop and work to a vision supported by their regional office. This approach was patchy.
- There was no automatic medical involvement and few PG deaneries or other doctors in education or management were involved. MADEL and SIFT operated in most places independently of consortia. Exceptions were in North Thames and the North West where regional directors of education and training with a multidisciplinary remit ensured better connections were made.
- Consortia were relatively small (over 40 initially), had middle level managers supported by chairs who were either full time NHS managers or non-executives. Initially they had infrastructure budgets of about £75 000, wholly insufficient to support what was quite a sophisticated management concept.
- They were not legal entities and depended on one of their statutory members managing finance and personnel and the legally binding contracts with higher education.
- Higher education providers were not allowed to become consortium members, thus keeping the level of relationship with them on a purchaser–provider basis rather than one of mutual understanding and partnership. Relationships with education could easily become fraught.
- Other non-NHS employers were never successfully engaged.

Those that worked well did so almost in spite of the formal system, realising that much of the important work lay outside the strict confines of the system.

It was hardly surprising that when the whole NHS education and training system was reviewed it was found to be fragmented and in many aspects not properly fit for purpose in a service needing to move towards a more integrated team-based approach with flexibility around functions determined by training and competence rather than just historical precedent. The review *A Health Service of all the Talents*[3] was stimulated by a report on workforce by the Health Select Committee in 1999. It came out in 2000 just before the *NHS Plan*[4] was published and became in effect the workforce blueprint for the *NHS Plan*. The main recommendations were:

- development of consortia into WDCs, which would be fewer in number, with higher level management, led by chief executives of NHS trust chief executive seniority and with a proper management infrastructure to support the work of the collaborative
- membership would include not only those who should have been in the consortium (i.e. both NHS and non-NHS employers), but also education providers, both higher and further education, and PG medical and dental education through the deaneries. As medical schools would be included, all aspects of medical education were to be involved
- The three existing education levies would lie within a single multiprofessional education and training levy (MPET) but would initially continue to exist in separate streams. In time all would be channelled through the WDC.

Twenty-seven confederations came into existence within a year of the report, in April 2001. From April 2002 all the MPET streams flowed through them, bringing the PG deaneries within their financial orbit. The concurrent development of strategic health authorities (28), which now provide the statutory base for the WDCs, and the slimming down of regional offices into four directorates of health and social care (DHSCs) has established a new direction of travel which you in the deaneries must watch and work around. This process was called 'shifting the balance of power'. However, many far less polite versions of the acronym StBoP exist! I will leave you to work out a few of your own. The rhetoric is devolution, but what is the reality? Have we seen the end of central command and control and micro management by ministers and the Department of Health?

This is the world which you now inhabit and in which you must develop relationships with the rest of the workforce development system. The current system is summarised in the following boxes, starting in Figure 10.1 with a diagrammatic overview of the workforce arrangements both nationally and locally. The boxes that follow Figure 10.1 give brief explanations of the organisations shown.

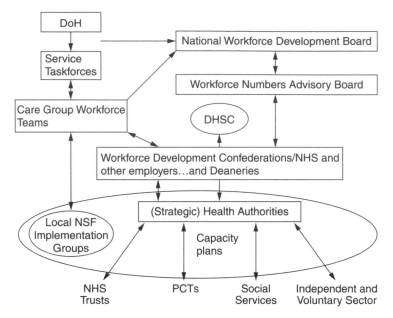

Figure 10.1 Proposed workforce planning arrangements.

National Workforce Development Board

- Set the strategic direction for workforce development.
- Ensure that a coherent and modernised pattern of workforce development is adopted throughout the NHS.

Care Group Workforce Teams

- Focus on workforce requirements for specific care groups.
- Take a national view on workforce development issues in their area.
- Identify workforce and education changes that are needed.
- Make recommendations on staffing requirements for their area.

Workforce Numbers Advisory Board

- Make recommendations on undergraduate and postgraduate training commissions for each group.
- Draw on recommendations from confederations and care group workforce teams.
- Look at requirements across all healthcare professions.

Health Communities

- All organisations will develop proper workforce plans supporting the HImP.
- Health authorities responsible for development and implementation of workforce capacity plans through PCTs.
- DHSCs performance manage health authorities (HAs) to ensure this happens.

Workforce Development Confederations

- Bring together NHS and non-NHS to plan the whole healthcare workforce.
- Work closely with Higher Education Institutions (HEIs), Learning and Skills Councils, and deaneries.
- Drive change in the way in which staff are educated, trained and employed.
- Develop comprehensive plans for delivering the workforce in their area.

Strategic Health Authorities (StHAs)

- Provide strategic direction.
- Performance manage PCTs and NHS trusts to ensure delivery of the *NHS Plan*, including workforce development issues.
- Develop capacity/improve services.

NHS Trusts

- Will continue to provide most secondary care and specialist services, working within delivery agreement with PCTs.
- Will devolve greater responsibility to clinical teams and foster the growth of clinical networks across NHS organisations.

Primary Care Trusts (PCTs)

- Lead NHS organisations in accessing need, planning and securing all health services and improving health.
- Lead on the development of all primary care services linked to local workforce development requirements.

The concept of a confederation and the implications for postgraduate deaneries

There is widespread misunderstanding about what a confederation is and should be. People constantly refer to confederations as if they are distinct entities to which workforce and education responsibility can be handed or who have to be worked with. You all do this. Yet the confederation is exactly what it says, a confederation of member organisations with a collective responsibility for local workforce and education issues. The deanery is part of this confederation. The confederation as a membership organisation must be distinguished from the confederation executive team headed by the chief executive, which exists to carry out the business and provide support and external linkages for the confederation membership. It is not an easy concept, especially in an NHS and education sector focused on individual organisations. Try substituting for 'The confederation needs to do this, we must work together to achieve this, it is our joint responsibility' and you begin to see the difference.

What does this mean as a GP director within your area of general practice and primary care? You are part of the deanery with responsibility for PG and continuing GP education and development, accountable to the WDC collective as one of its members and to the chief executives for the expenditure of MADEL, which comes through the WDC. You are accountable to the PG dean for the quality of your work and that of your GP team. You will have a responsibility to the Joint Committee on Postgraduate Training for General Practice (JCPTGP) and in the future to the Postgraduate Medical Education and Training Board for the quality of training, as well as to the GMC and possibly your local university. However, within the WDC, as part of a member organisation, you have scope to develop working relationships with the other members with a primary care interest, notably the PCTs, among which will be teaching PCTs. Remember they too will be new to all this and, because of the history of separation between the worlds of Hospital and Community Health Services (HCHS) and GMS, less familiar and less well founded in terms of education funding than their secondary care-based members of the WDC.

Primary care faces real challenges in terms of recruitment and retention of GPs and other clinical professional practice staff and their continuing development. If we go on working in the way that we do now it is likely that we will not be able to recruit sufficient skilled staff to cope. There is therefore going to have to be a fairly radical look at the way services are provided and staff are used, which is going to cut across the primary/secondary and the health/social care divides. Local health economies should be at the centre of the strategic thinking that underpins this. The last budget provided 44% growth in real terms for the NHS over the next five years. Expectations of service delivery will rise accordingly. The future NHS workforce and its capacity to work flexibly and imaginatively to deliver on issues of access to services, patient choice and the speed and quality of care has become the single most important determinant of success or failure of the NHS.

I believe that PG deaneries have a clear choice: to be part of the problem or part of the solution; to be part of a culture which complains about how terrible everything is with overwork, bureaucracy and endless targets, or to take the opportunity that some of these locally-based structures provide to supply clinical leadership and be part of preparing and supporting clinical professionals in a revamping of services. The latter will mean thinking about how your networks can interact with the PCTs and with higher and further education. Does your GP education experience have something to contribute to thinking about primary care more widely? Is the future one where you will seek to influence this broader agenda or do you think it best to focus on what you know? What is the future of primary care? What role can you as educationalists play in tackling the malaise and loss of confidence within clinical professions (not just medicine) whose implicit 'contract with society', built up throughout the twentieth century, is breaking down. This is not just abstract musing, but lies at the heart of the current recruitment and retention problem.

In Figure 10.1 the tradition has been a top-down one with the national driving the local. I think this now needs to be turned on its head with the local systems, as represented by strategic health authorities, PCTs and WDCs, driving the workforce development agenda and national systems to avoid omission and duplication, and to handle the management of those small specialist groups of staff whose numbers are too low for any local approach to be effective. In medicine the various top-down processes have failed consistently to deliver the right answer in relation to the medical workforce. There is no reason to believe that this will ever change. Local situations need local approaches with a sensitive national steer, not the current 'one size fits all' dogma which no-one owns.

If there is to be effective local leadership within an overall national vision, clinicians and managers have to come together so that the clinicians of tomorrow are no longer trained for yesterday's world. We need education (preparation for an unknown future) to be better balanced with training (preparation for a known future). Why not start with the WDC concept, an umbrella organisation within which collaboration and understanding between education and service can be explored for the benefit of the future provision of healthcare. How can you as influential GPs help that to happen?

'O that a man's reach should exceed his grasp, or what's a heaven for?' As GP leaders there is an opportunity to think a little about reach as well as the everyday business of grasp.

References

1 Department of Health (1989) *Working for Patients*. HMSO, London.

2 NHS Executive (1995) *Executive Letter (EL) (95) 27 – Education and Training in the New NHS*. NHS Executive, Leeds.

3 Department of Health (2000) *A Health Service of all the Talents: developing the NHS workforce*. Consultation document on the review of workforce planning. Department of Health, London.

4 Secretary of State for Health (2000) *The NHS Plan: a plan for investment, a plan for reform*. Department of Health, London.

CHAPTER 11

Whither the GP tutor?

John Howard

General practice tutors are at a critical stage of development. England and Wales have had a system of GP tutors for many years, organised and funded through deaneries from MADEL. The network of GP tutors was formalised and remunerated after the introduction of the PGEA in the 1990 Contract in England, Wales and Northern Ireland.[1] The situation has always been different in Scotland where no funding has been identified for such a network.

Tutors were originally introduced to provide continuing medical education for GP principals and retained doctors. However, they rapidly took responsibility for facilitating CPD, a much wider agenda, and one which involved interprofessional education and networking. They are now usually known as primary care or CPD tutors, reflecting their wider portfolio; some are not medically qualified. Tutors' roles have evolved rapidly in response to the needs of their local area. As a consequence, there is considerable variation between deaneries and PCOs in job descriptions, rates of pay and working practices.[2]

The introduction of appraisals, provided independently by PCOs under their clinical governance responsibilities, has generated further uncertainty.[3] Tutors have previously taken responsibility for the learning of individual GPs or their practices, often acting as mentors. However the appraisal scheme is formative and constructs a personal learning plan for all principals, with contact from the appraiser during the year of the plan. The task is exactly that which tutors have previously stated to be their own. The core functions of tutors are therefore unclear.

One way to clarify the situation is to reformulate uncertainty into a series of questions for discussion. The following issues reflect the uncertainty relating to management structures and role felt by tutors and their deaneries.

Questions of structure

- What should be the relationship between CPD tutors and PCOs?
- What should be the relationship between PCOs and confederations?

> • Do tutors need to be aligned with PCOs and perhaps higher education institutions?

Questions of process

- What is the role of CPD tutors now?
- What is the relationship between CPD tutors and appraisers?
- How should the quality assurance of appraisals be organised?
- What is the relationship between PGEA and appraisals, and personal learning and practice development plans and appraisals?

Questions of structure

What should be the management and accountability arrangements for CPD tutors?

In 1997 there were approximately 600 GP tutors.[4] It is more difficult to be exact about the number working now as some PCOs have apparently employed their own educationalists. Many CPD tutors remain part of the deanery structure, and are responsible to the regional director via a local AD. Other CPD tutors work in PCOs, with either shared employment between the deanery structure and a PCO, or employment solely by the PCO.

Given the uncertainty around place of employment and accountability, a brief and informal survey was undertaken at the 2002 UKCEA conference of half of the UK's deaneries, and provides a snapshot of the current situation. The results are shown in Table 11.1. The numbers relate to numbers of tutors, not sessions worked and are approximate as the survey was undertaken informally without preparation.

Altogether 11 deaneries were represented reporting on 235 tutors, 40% of the total number when surveyed in 1997.

If these figures are representative of the whole country, 64% (150) of tutors are solely employed and accountable to deaneries.

Thirty-six percent (85) of tutors have mixed employment status, being employed jointly by deaneries and trusts. However only 12.3% had shared accountability, and no deanery volunteered information about tutors employed and accountable solely within trusts. A more formal study of PCTs is necessary to establish whether tutors both employed by and accountable to trusts are present in the UK. However, this brief survey suggests that around

Table 11.1 Employment and accountability arrangements for CPD tutors

Deanery	Number of tutors	Employment	Accountability
W Scotland	23	Trust/deanery	Deanery
Sheffield	9	Trust/deanery	Trust/deanery
	10	Deanery	Deanery
N Ireland	10	Deanery	Deanery
North West	25	Deanery	Deanery
	5	Trust/deanery	Trust/deanery
Eastern	35	Deanery	Deanery
	15	Trust/deanery	Trust/deanery
Trent	15	Trust/deanery	Deanery
Wessex	12	Deanery	Deanery
London	40	Deanery	Deanery
	6	Trust/deanery	Deanery
Oxford	15	Trust/deanery	Deanery
	10	Various	Various
NE Scotland	4	Deanery	Deanery
Mersey	14	Deanery	Deanery
	2	Trust/deanery	Deanery

90% of tutors are fully accountable to deaneries no matter where they are employed, indicating perhaps the importance attached by directors to the maintenance of the CPD tutor network within the educational infrastructure.

The Kennedy report highlighted the importance of leadership and of effective CPD for all;[5] the past role of tutors through deaneries matches the recommendations exactly. It would seem that senior GP educators believe that educational leadership should come from an intact tutor network accountable to deaneries, which would accord with the Kennedy report recommendations. The need for local educators to interface effectively within PCTs makes joint appointments attractive. Because of the variations in local circumstances, the model of a joint appointment with PCTs may not always be appropriate, but it appears to be becoming more frequent. The possibility of tutors being employed directly by universities, a past suggestion, seemed to be less favoured in practice.

Some deaneries have banned tutors from taking up formal positions within PCOs. They felt it was difficult to delineate the work undertaken within each post and were concerned that the tutor may be paid twice for the same work. The majority of deaneries were not concerned about this and felt robust management arrangements were adequate to prevent this difficulty. Many

deaneries suggest tutors have over-performed compared to contracted expectations; current rates of pay did not adequately remunerate tutors and the better
rewarded jobs in PCOs were an attraction to a highly skilled workforce. It was
important to secure adequate future remuneration and conditions, a task that
COGPED and the GPC of the BMA must take seriously.

Questions of process

How should CPD be managed, given the proposed new contract for GPs and the new appraisal system? What should be the role of CPD tutors in the future ?

Because of the variations in local circumstances, it has almost become impossible to write a standard job description for CPD tutors; it has been simpler to
write a menu of possible activities dependent on perceived need. The National
Association of Primary Care Educators produced such a menu in 2000.[2] This
was written before the inauguration of PCTs in England and the introduction
of the appraisal scheme for principals. Tutors have continued to state that they
consider their primary role to be the support of learning for individual practitioners. This menu of possible activities is as follows:

- the management of PG learning, and the management of developmental
  change for practitioners and local PCO(s) on behalf of the DPGPE
- a mentoring system, either for practices or individuals, promoting lifelong
  learning
- educational support to individuals and practices, including the implementation of assessment and appraisal tools
- the assessment, licensing and certification on behalf of the director of uni-
  or multiprofessional educational activities provided for general practice in
  the locality
- continuing medical education (CME) – ensuring provision of learning activities, courses and schemes; not necessarily provided directly by the tutor
- the promotion of multiprofessional audit and clinical guidelines with other
  involved agencies
- an involvement in the locality educational strategic development with secondary care
- networking with stakeholders in primary care and higher education
- resource location to support learning in primary care

- advising on the organisation and culture in PCOs
- the promotion of Postgraduate Medical Centres (PGMCs) as a resource for learning.

The creation of clinical governance as a mechanism to perfomance-manage CPD for individuals and teams has altered the balance of need for educational expertise. Whereas in the past the CPD tutor, usually working outside the PCO, has been the acknowledged developer of CPD strategy, deliverer of provision, assessor of quality and purveyor of credits arising from CPD, clinical governance places the functions of the CPD tutor at the centre of the local PCO stage. There must therefore be more integrated working between tutors and PCOs.

The appraisal system reflects this need for educational skills. Training for appraisers has been provided by the government for one year only, and no specific educational support or quality assurance mechanisms have been specified. PCOs will need to develop both of these functions for appraisal to be a success; the skills and networks of deanery tutors are well suited to these tasks.

A further important requirement arising from the appraisal system will be the delivery of targeted continuing medical education specified in personal and practice professional development plans. The appraisal system will for many provide, for the first time, the collation of learning needs for the professionals working in a trust. If these learning needs are not met, the system will rapidly be discredited. Tutors will have an important role in meeting these needs.

The suggested contact between appraiser and GP is not thought to be long enough for an effective personal learning plan to be both developed and carried through. It is likely that many GPs will continue to use their local tutor for advice on needs assessment, the construction of their plan, and implementation issues between appraisals. The ratio of tutors to GPs has been far too small to allow proper support for GPs in the past, and the employment of appraisers will help this problem. Tutors may as a result be able to work with clinical governance leads to assist practices in both compiling and implementing practice professional development plans. The relationship between the tutor and the PCT is therefore very important. Suggestions for educational roles for trust board members were set out in *Vision 2000* and have changed relatively little since then.[2]

Quality assurance and support of appraisers may become a deanery function. Oxford has telephone support for appraisers from associate advisers,[6] but other areas are devolving this to tutors. How quality assurance would work is not clear, and most PCOs are not ready for this development as yet.

The proposed new contract for GPs will see the end of the PGEA, perhaps to be replaced by funding for personal learning plans and a system of career development involving skills, special interest and leadership training.[7] It is likely that courses appropriate for CPD will continue to need certification through the network of tutors to ensure NHS resources are directed at appropriate developments. This mechanism should also be used to encourage interprofessional learning, another key recommendation of the Kennedy report.[5] A longer-term aim for the certification of CPD should be to deliver academic accreditation for PG courses and learning; tutors' links to deaneries may be important in this context.

Perhaps the most important function for tutors is educational leadership. Since the Chief Medical Officer's report on CPD[8] it has been accepted that inputs to CPD should come from both the service and the individual. The mechanism for individual professionals to feed service needs to those developing strategy in health authorities has not been present in the past. CPD tutors will be in possession of aggregated learning needs for the local professionals if their integration with PCOs is effective. They will, as a group in a deanery, be able to feed these needs to WDCs as a CPD strategy document.

Conclusions

When we reconsider the questions posed earlier in this chapter, a new list of core tasks emerges for the future CPD tutor, those of:

- educational leadership – producing a strategy document for WDCs
- supporting and training appraisers
- CME provision derived from aggregated learning needs
- CPD support and facilitation, including the encouragement of inter-professional education
- the certification of appropriate courses and learning
- networking locally and within the deanery, both within and outside the discipline.

Our next step is to meet this challenge.

References

1 Department of Health (1989) *General Practice in the National Health Service; 1990 contract.* HMSO, London.

2 National Association of Primary Care Educators (NAPCE) (2000) *Vision 2000 – managed CPD in the new NHS.* NAPCE, Manchester.

3 Department of Health (2002) *Appraisal for General Practitioners Working in the NHS.* (www.doh.gov.uk/gpappraisal)

4 *National Association of Primary Care Educators Survey* (1997) Unpublished.

5 Bristol Royal Infirmary (2001) *The Final Report of the Bristol Royal Infirmary Inquiry.* (www.bristol-inquiry.org.uk)

6 Dr Richard Flew, Oxford Deanery. Personal communication.

7 BMA (2002) *Your Contract, Your Future.* General Practitioners Committee, BMA, London.

8 Chief Medical Officer, Department of Health (1998) *A Review of CPD in General Practice.* Department of Health, London.

Based on a workshop given at the 2002 UKCEA conference. With thanks to the workshop members Drs Stuart Murray, Pat Lane, Dr Arthur Hibble, Julia Whiteman, Malcom Valentine, Kevin Ilsley, Terry Bradley, Richard Flew, Dr Robin While, Dr Neil Jackson.

CHAPTER 12

Continuing professional development for remote and rural GPs – the role of telemedicine

Stewart Wilkie

Telemedicine is the provision of healthcare and education using telecommunication networks. It is a generic term that covers diagnosis and treatment of patients as well as education in healthcare. The term 'videoconferencing' can be used synonymously to describe a meeting between two or more sites using telemedicine equipment to provide video and audio communication. In the UK, telemedicine has been used successfully in several clinical fields including dermatology and cardiology and it is increasingly used in education.[1,2] CME and CPD are important for all medical practitioners particularly with the introduction of appraisal and revalidation. For those that are isolated by geographical barriers the opportunity to participate in organised educational events can be limited.

The use of videoconferencing in continuing GP education was debated at the UKCEA conference 2002. Delegates took part in a videoconference using a standard stand-alone system at ISDN 2 – a relatively low bandwidth. The quality of interaction was generally agreed to be excellent and many of the following points were highlighted at the workshop.

Telemedicine and rural general practice

The use of telemedicine equipment for videoconferencing can improve access to education irrespective of distance and perhaps can been seen as most useful in remote areas or areas where travel is time-consuming and difficult. The terms 'rural' and 'remote' are difficult to define. There are many areas in the UK that can be described as rural and this is particularly obvious in Scotland. The Scottish Executive has used a working definition of rural as an area with a population density of less than one person per hectare.[3] Using this definition, 89% of Scotland's landmass and 29% of its population can be described as rural. People living in rural areas express high rates of satisfaction with GP services (80–89%) and perceive these services as vital to maintaining a thriving community.[4] GPs working in remote island areas of Scotland, perhaps the most geographically isolated group in the UK, feel that the advantages of practising in such areas outweigh the disadvantages. Despite this there are major problems with GP principal and registrar recruitment in these areas. Ross and Gillies (1999) found that professional isolation, heavy clinical responsibility and onerous on-call commitments deterred applicants for these posts.[5] GPs in these rural areas are less likely to attend PG educational meetings than their colleagues in urban areas.[6] Telemedicine is not a substitute for conventional consultations and educational events. It is however a useful addition that can increase educational opportunities for GPs in rural areas,[7] help reduce feelings of isolation and may help to make such posts more attractive.

Telemedicine for technophobes

Videoconferencing allows users to take part in meetings despite being geographically remote. The technology behind videoconferencing is rapidly changing and the quality of the audio and video equipment is now excellent and affordable. Good quality stand-alone systems can be bought for £2000 to £5000 and personal computer (PC)-based systems cost less than half that. There still exists a tremendous amount of jargon and technical detail relating to telemedicine that is used by IT enthusiasts. This only serves to confuse and put potential users off. Using telemedicine equipment is no more difficult than using a home video recorder. It is certainly well within the grasp of all medical practitioners. A straightforward account of the jargon and the system is all that is needed to demystify videoconferencing and this is outlined below.

Components of a videoconferencing network

A simple videoconferencing network can be purchased as a stand-alone system or it can be incorporated into an existing computer system. Irrespective of the type of system the hardware consists of three main parts: the input device, the codec and the output device.

Input device (e.g. microphone, camera, document camera, laptops)

This is required to provide the visual picture and the audio that is transmitted to the remote site. The quality of the video that is sent can be affected greatly by the quality of the lens or camera that is connected to the system. Most stand-alone systems come with an inbuilt camera and attached room microphone. Add-on equipment can enhance the educational use of videoconferencing equipment. Document cameras can be used like a traditional overhead projector to provide the remote site with an image of any object placed on it. Standard laptop computers can be connected to transmit computer slide-show presentations to participants.

Codec (coding–decoding) equipment

This provides the analogue to digital interface for the input device. It also does all the clever things like signal processing, and acts as the digital to analogue interface for the output device. The codec is not something that most users need to worry about too much.

Output device (e.g. TV, video monitor, loudspeakers)

In most systems the output device will be an ordinary TV or computer monitor. Most stand-alone systems allow a data projector to be connected and this can be used to project the video output onto a projector screen. This can be useful if there are larger groups of participants present.

Videoconferences may be linked-up 'point-to-point' (i.e. a single site communicates with one other site) or via a multipoint control unit (MCU) or 'bridge'. A bridge enables more than two sites to link up simultaneously in a 'multiconference'. In addition to the hardware, the data must be transmitted between the connected sites. At present there are essentially two main methods of doing this:

- ISDN technology
- the internet (virtual private network)(VPN).

ISDN (integrated services digital network)

Videoconferencing units are commonly connected via ISDN lines. These are essentially telephone lines that handle information in a digital manner and much more quickly than older analogue telephone equipment. ISDN lines use digital signals to transmit voice, video and data. The type of ISDN line installed determines the amount of data that can be transmitted. Each ISDN line has two channels (ISDN 2) that can each transmit 64 kilobits of information per second (kbps). In practice smooth video and audio transmission requires six ISDN channels (ISDN 6) although if the user is skilled in teaching over a video-conferencing system, ISDN 2 can suffice. There are benefits and disadvantages with ISDN:

Benefits
- it is a reliable technology
- ISDN is the most widely used method of videoconferencing
- the system is internationally compatible
- ISDN networks follow the existing telecommunication infrastructure
- the bandwidth has guaranteed performance.

Disadvantages
- call charges can be expensive and are determined by the number of ISDN lines used
- ISDN connections are currently unavailable in many rural areas.

Virtual private network

A VPN is a private connection between two computers, videoconferencing systems or networks over a shared or public network. In practical terms users are connected to each other via the internet, using internet protocol (IP) rather than relying on the more expensive ISDN system. If the internet is used for videoconferencing over long distances, then the need to purchase expensive leased lines is avoided, as are expensive long distance call charges on ISDN calls between distant sites. Instead the call is simply connected locally to the internet service provider (ISP) and calls are charged at local rates.

The benefits of using IP for videoconferencing include:

- the internet is now widely accessible to most people
- in many cases existing telecommunication lines may be used
- call charges made using IP are significantly less than ISDN.

There are some drawbacks of using IP for videoconferencing. These include:

- concerns over compatibility issues
- quality of service is not guaranteed
- information transmitted over the internet must be dealt with securely and security issues can incur further expense and complexity.

Telemedicine can be performed in 'real time' or by using pre-recorded material, much like a television broadcast. Real-time interactive video meetings are arguably the most suitable format for medical education meetings and have been shown to be effective.[8]

The use of telemedicine in education

Distance learning using telemedicine is not a new concept. The early adopters of the technology were those industrialised countries with large rural areas of land such as Australia, Canada and Norway – indeed telemedicine has been used since the late 1980s in Norway.[9] In the UK the use of telemedicine is not yet widespread although a number of projects have explored the use of telemedicine for distance education as well as clinical uses. Teaching sessions have been conducted with foreign sites[10] and cardiopulmonary resuscitation training[11] and nurse education has also been provided this way.[12] From a technological point of view, the equipment has improved tremendously and the jerky, poor-quality images that were a feature of early systems are now a thing of the past.

There are many advantages to providing CME to remote users in this way:

- participants do not have to travel large distances to meet their educational needs
- a specialist can address many sites at the same time
- the session is interactive and participants can get immediate feedback
- it can reduce professional isolation.

The process of delivering an educational programme using telemedicine differs slightly from conventional educational meetings and some important points should be followed. Participants should be aware of the need to speak clearly and users must be familiar with the equipment.[13] Unlike conventional television broadcasts where the complete scene is continuously renewed or 're-freshed', it is only those parts of the image which have moved that are refreshed in a telemedicine conference. Excessive movement can lead to a reduction in image quality when connected at lower ISDN rates. Presenters should move and gesture smoothly to minimise this. This is not a problem when connected at data rates of ISDN 6 and above. Educational materials should be prepared in advance and the appropriate font size, colour and layout should be used if a computer slide-show is incorporated. Taking part in videoconferences can be demanding and adult learning and group facilitation principles should be applied to maintain the interest of participants and to ensure that educational objectives are met.[14]

Conclusion

There are a number of telemedicine projects in the UK at present and although it is the clinical uses of telemedicine that are perhaps most obvious, it is equally important to consider the educational needs of rural GPs as this directly impacts on rural health. Strong support and a sound infrastructure are needed to implement these projects successfully and thorough evaluation is required. In those parts of the country where professional and geographical isolation present everyday barriers to education for rural GPs, the potential benefit and role of telemedicine is clear.

References

1   Loane MA, Bloomer SE, Corbett R *et al.* (2001) A randomized controlled trial assessing the health economics of realtime teledermatology compared with conventional care: an urban versus rural perspective. *J Telemed Telecare.* **7**: 101–18.

2   Shanit D, Cheng A and Greenbaum RA (1996) Telecardiology: supporting the decision-making process in general practice. *J Telemed Telecare.* **2**: 7–13.

3   Randall JN (1985) Economic trends and support to economic activity in rural Scotland. *Scottish Economic Bulletin.* **31**: 10–20.

4   Hope S, Anderson S and Sawyer B (2000) *The Quality of Services in Rural Scotland.* Scottish Executive Central Research Council. HMSO, London.

5   Ross S and Gillies JCM (1999) Characteristics and career intentions of Scottish rural and urban GP registrars: cause for concern? *Health Bull.* **57**: 44–52.

6   Murray TS, Dyker GS, Kelly MH *et al.* (1993) Demographic characteristics of general practitioners attending educational meetings. *Br J Gen Pract.* **43**: 467–9.

7   Callas PW, Ricci MA and Caputo MP (2000) Improved rural access to continuing medical education through interactive videoconferencing. *Telemed J E-Health.* **6**: 393–9.

8   Hampton CL, Mazmanian PE and Smith TJ (1994) The interactive videoconference: an effective CME delivery system. *J Contin Educ Health Prof.* **14**: 83–9.

9   Elford DR (1997). Telemedicine in northern Norway. *J Telemed Telecare.* **3**: 1–22.

10 Brebner EM, Brebner JA, Norman JN *et al.* (1997) Intercontinental postmortem studies using interactive television. *J Telemed Telecare.* **3**: 48–52.

11 Atkinson PRT, Bingham J, McNicholl BP *et al.* (1999) Telemedicine and cardiopulmonary resuscitation: the value of video-link and telephone instruction to a mock bystander. *J Telemed Telecare.* **5**: 242–5.

12 Jarrett C, Wainwright P and Lewis L (1997) Education and training of practice nurses. *J Telemed Telecare.* **3**: 40–2.

13 Sengupta TK, Wallace DA, Clark SL and Bannan G (1998) Videoconferencing: practical advice on implementation. *Aust J Rural Health.* **6**: 2–4.

14 Kaufman DM and Brock H (1998) Enhancing interaction using videoconferencing in continuing health education. *J Contin Educ Health Prof.* **18**: 81–5.

Based on a workshop at the 2002 UKCEA conference. With thanks to the workshop participants for their valuable contributions Drs Reed Bowden, Mike Grenville, Kevin Ilsley, Neil Jackson, Anthea Lints, Professor Stuart Murray, Steve Vincent and also to Dr Linda Hislop for co-ordinating the videoconference.

CHAPTER 13

Accredited professional development

Peter Jenkins and Karen Finlay

This chapter, and the workshop on which it is based, shares the experiences of the accredited professional development (APD) programme, which was piloted by the KSS Deanery in 2001, working in conjunction with the RCGP.

Background to APD

The aim of CME is to sustain the professional development of GPs and help them to provide high-quality patient care throughout their career, and to keep up to date with developments in general practice. The APD programme and resource materials were initially developed by Professors Dame Lesley Southgate and Janet Grant.

What is APD?

The APD programme is designed as a new approach to CPD, to offer ongoing support as GPs – principals or non-principals – continue their professional development as part of their everyday practice. The APD process is a semi-structured process that will help GPs to collect all the information and evidence that will be required for annual appraisals and revalidation, over a five-year period. The structure of the APD programme is to encourage learning that is relevant to the individual's everyday needs and practice, it is highly relevant and well focused on the day to day work of the average GP. This programme will allow GPs to plan their learning, demonstrate the quality of their practice as they continue to look after their patients, and also provide a simple means of providing evidence and documentation which will be useful for appraisals and revalidation in the future.

How does it work?

The APD programme is based on *Good Medical Practice* as published by the GMC.[1,2] It consists of six modules spread over five years, and a formal annual peer review meeting with a trained facilitator.

The ongoing module:
- keeping up to date and improving care.

This is a continuous module over the five years that allows the individual to identify areas of practice that require updating and improving, and encourages the participants to carry out educational activities to fulfil those learning needs.

Five stand-alone modules are available; these can be rotated throughout the five year programme. GPs will choose when and how often to undertake each module; it is recommended that each is undertaken once every five years, in order to ensure that the full evidence is available for revalidation.

The other five modules are:
- communication skills
- record keeping
- access and team working
- referrals and prescribing
- complaints and removals.

The APD facilitator

Each GP will be allocated to an APD facilitator, who will encourage the participating GPs to identify and prioritise their educational needs based on their everyday experience. Contact with the facilitator will be provided throughout the year, either by email, phone, mail, or it may prove beneficial to work with colleagues or friends in the form of a local APD group. The facilitator and the participant will meet at least once a year for a professional review, the APD folder will be reviewed and, in a confidential setting, areas of strengths, weaknesses, and areas to be concentrated on in the coming year will be discussed. The APD facilitators will participate in regular training and support schemes, they will have a good knowledge of the principles of adult education, be skilled in giving feedback, and guiding individuals to identify their own learning needs.

The process of APD incorporates all stages of the educational cycle, namely identifying learning needs, recording baseline knowledge, fulfilling those learning needs, evaluating that learning, and applying the new knowledge in everyday work. The individuals in turn may want to share their new knowledge with other members of their team or other colleagues.

Documentation provided

The participant will be provided with forms to demonstrate their learning and progress; there is a form to fill in with the completion of personal and professional details, diary sheets to complete as a record of learning on a regular basis, record sheets for the ongoing module, and record sheets for the five individual modules. Each applicant is provided with a resource file, which contains a framework for each module, and ideas on how they may wish to approach the topic and carry out that module, but these ideas are not exclusive and are only suggestions.

Strengths of the APD process

One of the main strengths of the APD process is that it is very personal and individual, and participants can include work that they are carrying out for other reasons or other areas of study, as there will be much relevant common ground. Participants will be able to include any other work they are doing towards other quality awards as designed by the RCGP. There is flexibility in the system so each individual GP will be able to develop special interests, or include practice-based activities.

Context of APD

All doctors will be required to demonstrate on a regular basis that they are fit to continue to practise. The introduction of revalidation has been designed to demonstrate to the public that doctors provide a high standard of care, to promote high standards across the medical profession, and to identify doctors who may need early support or education. The APD process has been designed to help the participating GP to document and demonstrate, with evidence, that they are following a continuous learning programme, in order to achieve high standards of care. It is envisaged that the APD folder could be submitted as part of the revalidation portfolio.

Pilot programme in KSS Deanery

This programme was piloted by KSS Deanery in 2001, 200 participants were included in the pilot, 35 facilitators were trained – all either GP tutors or course organisers, so they had knowledge of GP education. One hundred and eight participants completed the programme in the year. The feedback from the participants was positive, it was viewed as user-friendly, practice-based, highly relevant, yet could be tailor-made to meet the individual's needs. The resource pack was invaluable, and gave ideas on specific tools that could be used, for example rating scales, PUNs and DENs, significant event analysis (SEA), peer observation and skills assessment techniques. The programme encouraged people to try out new skills, and develop existing skills.

Further information

Full details of the APD programme can be obtained from the RCGP.

References

1   Royal College of General Practitioners and General Practitioners Committee (2002) *Good Medical Practice for General Practitioners*. RCGP/GPC, London.

2   General Medical Council (2001) *Good Medical Practice*. GMC, London.

CHAPTER 14

GP appraisals and revalidation – the role of the educationalist

Alex Trompetas

From 2002–2003 PCTs will be responsible for arranging annual appraisals for GPs in their area. To meet this requirement, a rolling national programme of appraiser training has been instigated with around 800 GP appraisers trained in the first wave. The appraisal process will involve a one-to-one meeting between appraiser and appraisee and and examination of the appraisee's developmental needs structured around a PDP. In preparation for the appraisal, GPs will collate and review their educational activities for the year and formulate plans for future years. In addition to locally organised annual appraisal, there will be an external revalidation visit every five years. The details of the mechanism of revalidation are still to be finalised but it is clear that the annual appraisal and PDP will form an essential part of this process.

Despite the fact that the appraisals process is to be led by PCTs, the Department of Health has emphasised the developmental nature of appraisal and its primary purpose of education, training and development as opposed to performance management.

With the arrival of GP appraisal, the following questions are raised for the managers and providers of medical education.

- What is the role of the primary care educationalist in the appraisal?
- How do we balance the educational and developmental aspect of appraisal against the background of performance management?
- What input and preparation can educators have in the pre-appraisal period?
- How do educators assist and help in the implementation and development of education needs and plans which arise as a result of appraisal?

Resources

Let us first examine the resourcing of educational support for appraisal. PCTs are required to fund the appraisal process from their existing annual allocations. The deaneries were granted a small amount of additional funding – rather late in the day – in October 2002. This money was specifically earmarked for appraisals but will not go far. Many PCTs around the country have already actively started the appraisal process and were following different models for appraisals and PDPs. Some PCTs were planning to appraise just a small proportion of their GPs during the first year, a strategy dictated mainly by financial considerations with priority given to GPs who were likely to be revalidated early because of their GMC registration number. Although the government initially suggested that all GP principals would be appraised by March 2003, a more realistic figure of 20% of GPs in the first year is used as a target by many PCTs. There are some common key themes emerging in geographically dispersed PCT areas. In London for example, attempts were made through a co-ordinating body, involving the chief executives for the different PCTs, to harmonise appraisal activity. More usually, the key personnel involved and organisation and development of the appraisals are vastly different in different areas.

With the evolution of such a multiplicity of different models, the GP educationalists need to help ensure a balance of the organisational development aspect of this process – with the inevitable performance implications – against an individual's training needs. GP appraisals and PDPs are seen as intricately linked. However, an organisation carrying out appraisals should be able to separate the educational process that drives the PDP from the governance initiatives that underpin performance management.

Much can be learned from the experience of GP vocational training, where, since the introduction of summative assessment, personal development and performance have been linked in one process during the GP registrar year. The trainer/registrar relationship is illustrative. In this teacher/learner relationship the same person, i.e. the trainer, is involved both in the performance assessment and the educational aspect of the personal development of the registrar. Thus both formative and summative assessment roles are present in the same relationship. The principle accepted in this instance by the educators involved in GP training is that assessment drives learning.

The role of the primary care tutor

A review of different experiences amongst primary care tutors, many of whom are former GP tutors, reveals that in different areas primary care tutors have different degrees of involvement in appraisals. In some areas primary care tutors are appraisers themselves, involved in hands-on appraisals, whereas in some areas they are more involved in the organisational aspects of appraisal working as PCT education leads or with PCT educational committees in setting up the appraisal system. Finally, in some PCTs, primary care tutors seem to be undertaking both roles, i.e. planning appraisals as well as doing them.

Other examples of primary care tutor involvement include such work as pre-appraisal support by primary care tutors for individual GPs. These GPs, once prepared, would then progress to have a formal appraisal with a trained appraiser. A similar post-appraisal model is suggested where primary care tutors working with PCTs will support GPs after their formal appraisal and help them develop some of the educational aspects of their PDP that may have arisen as a result of the appraisal.

The relationship between primary care tutors and PCTs is also very variable. It would appear that in some areas, deanery-employed educators are also employed by the local PCT. In some areas the primary care tutor is also head/director of education for the PCT in a directly employed role. Such relationships need to be examined to see if there are conflicts in the roles and responsibilities arising in working for the deanery and working for the PCT. It would also appear that one of the main areas where primary care educators were already involved nationwide with PCTs was in approving PDPs for educational content and recommending them to the relevant deanery for accreditation for PGEA.

Education versus performance management

Appraisals have been introduced against a background of performance management not only locally, with PDPs heavily influenced by local clinical governance needs, but also nationally through the link with revalidation. The relevance of revalidation to the introduction of appraisals needs to be considered and, in particular, the educational and personal development aspects of these processes.

What is the significance of setting standards for revalidation and what are the educational implications of developing the criteria by which these standards would be measured? Many educators believe that revalidation will stay constant with time in relation to its standards. However, these same educators also feel that what might change in time are the criteria used to measure these standards. These criteria may be influenced by the development of the GP medical workforce and the expectation that with suitable educational preparation, an increasing proportion of GPs will perform better against fixed measurable standards. The criteria for revalidation will also be affected by developments in medical knowledge, accepted group or peer practice and changes in the public's expectations of its GPs. It is speculated among educational circles therefore, that over a time span of 10–20 years, standards of good practice – already developed by relevant professional bodies – will remain constant, but the criteria used to measure these same standards may change.

Practical considerations

There is widespread agreement among deaneries around the country and a realisation among the personnel employed by these deaneries that primary care tutors need to work closely with PCTs and that each PCT should have substantial educationalist input. This input should come either from educationalists directly employed by PCTs and/or educationalists not employed by PCTs i.e. employed by deanery, medical school or other research and academic bodies.

The emergent teaching PCTs are providing excellent examples in leading the way in utilising educational resources and there are many other innovative ways of using primary care tutors developing around the country.

Finally it is evident that PCTs locally need vastly increased educational input and, therefore, an increased primary care educator role. There are some immediately implementable practical solutions to this problem. An increase in the local educational leadership in each area can be achieved by developing and appointing more educators, or increasing the time commitment of the currently appointed primary care tutors in order that they can become effectively involved in the appraisal process. Currently most primary care tutors in different areas are employed by the deanery for two sessions per week. Increasing the time commitment of existing primary care tutors may be an option for some primary care tutors but may not be possible for others. This is because some of the existing primary care tutors have time constraints. There is certainly an anxiety in primary care tutor circles that attempting to increase existing primary care tutor time commitments and duties may demoralise them and have the opposite effect.

An effective local implementation of GP appraisals with valid workable PDPs that will benefit the individuals and their PCTs needs to develop hand in hand with an educational strategy. Increased investment in time and resources is required and deaneries and PCTs should work together with the help of workforce confederations to achieve increased investment in primary care education in order to deliver appraisals and, at last, PDPs for all GPs.

Further reading

- Fletcher C (1997) *Appraisal* (2e). IPD, London.

- Fletcher C (2001) Performance appraisal and management: the developing research agenda. *J Occup Organis Psychol.* **74**: 473–87.

- NHS Modernisation Agency (2002) *Appraisals for General Practitioners.* Department of Health, London.

- NHS Modernisation Agency (2002) *Appraisals for General Practitioners, Training the Appraisers.* Department of Health, London.

- (www.doh.gov.uk/gpappraisal)

- (www.londondeanery.ac.uk/gp/home.htm) (vocational training menu and summative assessment)

Based on a workshop discussion at the 2002 UKCEA conference. With thanks to the workshop participants Drs Robin While, Terry Bradley, Richard Flew, Malcolm Lewis, Rob Caird, Guy Houghton, Adrian Ball, Steve Ball, Sylvia Chudley, Andrew Bailey, Bob Kirk.

CHAPTER 15

Using appreciative inquiry as a method of appraising the new GP retainer scheme

Rebecca Viney

As for the majority of chapters in this book, what follows is based on the proceedings of a workshop undertaken at the 2002 UKCEA conference. The difference here though is that we shall be examining both content and process, as this chapter takes us in two directions at the same time being both an exploration of the new GP retainer scheme and an exposition of the organisational tool of appreciative inquiry.

So what is appreciative inquiry?

Appreciative inquiry is an approach to thinking that works from the proposition of affirmative action and visions of the possible.[1] The alternative model is the critical analysis deficit model; the unfortunate side-effect of this approach is that we amplify the problems and keep finding more.

Appreciative inquiry has been used in a vast number of different situations. As part of organisational redesign, it has been used to identify and create an ideal environment for the development of success. The key is not to focus on saying what is wrong; rather, it is about focusing on the successful examples in the past and present. We build a picture of the themes and ideas that we know we can do, and that work. We develop an individual and collective mind-set of what we are capable of, that is grounded in reality. It is a definite shift from our traditions of education and training where the concentration is on what is wrong. When developing propositions and possibilities, appreciative inquiry envisages what might be (based on what is), and stimulates a dialogue on what should be, before finally focusing on what will be. By involving everyone's experience and energy in developing the themes and possibilities we have a greater chance of getting there.

Appreciative inquiry in action

Appreciative inquiry is based on dialogue. The first step is to collect opinions and observations of everyone involved through telling stories of what has been and is successful. These observations are then shared in a workshop format to identify the themes and topics that that run through the stories. Finally, a selection of the most important themes forms the basis for building a series of provocative propositions that describes how the organisation will be.

What has happened?

Six deans, deputy deans and associate deans who were responsible for running the GP retainer scheme in their deaneries met in a workshop at the 2002 UKCEA conference. Some had inherited the post and others had a long-standing interest in the GP retainer scheme. Success stories were encouraged and soon began to flow. Several themes emerged and a multitude of examples of success that I shall illustrate below.

Theme: educational opportunities

The discovery

> The new retainer scheme allows retainee GPs 28 hours of paid educational time. Practices continue to receive their payment of £53.80 per session for all kinds of leave including, education, annual, sick and maternity leave.[2]

We heard that allowing practices to receive payment for all leave sessions had allowed retainees to enjoy paid protected time to keep up to date and to address their CPD. It was noted that it was particularly important for retainees to study in paid time, as many retainees have to pay childcare costs out of taxed income in order to attend educational sessions.[3]

Some deaneries had facilitated the evolution of very popular learning groups, run for and by retainees.[4] In addition we heard that these were frequently funded by the deanery or PCT as well as being PGEA accredited. Others had set up interactive websites for their retainees to have a discussion forum. VTSs were also welcoming retainees to attend their meetings.

In the new scheme three hours of paid educational time is to be taken within the practice.

This development involves a variety of learning opportunities. For example, we heard that some educational supervisors facilitated personal learning plans, others provided mentorship on a weekly or monthly basis, and others included the retainee in practice educational meetings within paid time.

To facilitate retainees into mainstream education, a number of useful techniques had been employed. We heard that one deanery had held informal gatherings of PCT chairs with local educationalists at a well-known local watering hole and that this had built bridges. Retainees were presented as a valuable part of general practice who needed to be embraced into mainstream educational initiatives locally, as they had tended to be forgotten in the past.[5]

In the London Deanery, GP tutors for non-principals had been employed to facilitate retainees into mainstream education, to approve the personal learning plans, and to ensure that the retainees and educational supervisors were aware of and implementing the educational aspects of the scheme. In addition, residential meetings for tutors, programme directors and course organisers had been used to introduce the concept of generic education and lifelong learning for all GPs. Barriers were being dismantled and bridges were being built to include all GPs, whatever their contractual status, wherever education was provided locally.

We heard that the London Deanery had been encouraging retainees to become involved in teaching medical students and thereby introducing them into the educational circuit. They were able to do this in addition to their four clinical sessions. This has been warmly welcomed both by the retainees and the medical schools. Another deanery combined retainee meetings with local faculty meetings, which has resulted in local retainees being more involved in the faculty.

In London, retainees are also being actively encouraged to apply to be appraisers; this is seen as being of particular significance with the introduction of GP non-principal appraisal in April 2003.

The dream

The very best conditions based on best practice. What would it look like?

- Eight paid sessions for personal development
- Three hours of one-to-one mentorship by the practice educational facilitator, spread regularly throughout the year
- Self-directed learning groups in paid protected time
- A discussion forum for regional retainees on an interactive website

- IT training
- Opportunities to attend local VTS meetings
- Opportunities to receive mailings to local mainstream educational meetings
- Increased awareness of local funding streams for courses
- Appointment of tutors for non-principals to facilitate retainees into local initiatives, and assist with preparation for appraisal and PDPs
- Opportunities to teach medical students
- Links with the local faculty
- Retainees encouraged to become appraisers

Theme: assessment of practices

The discovery

The new scheme requires that practices be of training practice standard or on target to achieve these standards within a defined time frame.

Most areas had a surplus of practices seeking retainees, however this was not true of every area. We heard how new funding, earmarked to increase the number of training practices, had assisted practices who were stepping towards becoming retaining or training practices. It was noted that this had allowed more practices to become eligible to employ GPs on the retainer scheme. It was reflected that a great deal of work was involved in visiting practices that aspire to join the scheme. There was a variety of ways in which retaining practices were approved and reapproved. All deaneries visited first time practices if they were not already training practices. Thereafter a range of methods was used to check they were maintaining standards every three to five years. Practices are asked to write in to the deanery if they have undergone any major changes since their initial application.

The dream

The very best conditions based on best practice. What would it look like?

- All non-training practices are visited and a report written
- Practices are reapproved every 3–5 years depending on findings at the initial visit
- Practice informs deanery of any major changes which might affect the retainees, supervisor and/or conditions of employment

Theme: educational supervision

The discovery

It is a requirement that the educational supervisor is educationally trained.

In the London Deanery it had been found to be useful to have an application form, which specifically asks that the educational supervisor demonstrates their own CPD, as well as knowledge and experience in education. Appraisal of the retainee and educational supervisor at the annual reapplication by questionnaire highlighted most deficiencies so that they could be addressed. At least one deanery, Wessex, has provided a course starting for educational supervisors.[6]

The dream

The very best conditions based on best practice. What would it look like?

That the educational supervisor:

- is assessed for educational suitability initially
- is aware of scheme aims and responsibilities
- may attend training days.

Theme: exit strategy

The discovery

In the GP retainer scheme the retainer applies annually to stay on the scheme.

Although it is hoped that practices will take on their retainee as a partner or long-term assistant when they are no longer eligible for the scheme, in reality this does not often occur. In the fourth or fifth year some deaneries offer career counselling. It became apparent that finding suitable employment after the scheme was a problem for retainees. However despite there being many more salaried options available to GPs than in the past, these posts do not offer the flexibility, stability, terms and conditions or educational input that many women with young children seek. These doctors greatly value the educational component and the ability to tailor their work to their childcare needs that the retainer scheme can offer.

In November 2002 the Flexible Career Scheme for GPs was launched. It is designed to encourage practices to allow part-timers to work more flexibly, while allowing them good terms and conditions, using *Improving Working Lives* for guidance.[7] It is envisaged that this will be one of the routes that GPs wishing to work flexibly or part-time will choose to follow after or instead of the retainer scheme.

The dream

The very best conditions based on best practice. What would it look like?

An exit strategy will be assisted by:

- an annual PDP including an annual review of career plans
- a range of flexible employment opportunities with modern fair contracts for GPs wishing to work flexibly or part-time
- quality career counselling
- protected time for education being central to any future contracts.

Theme: terms and conditions

The discovery

Although deaneries do not have responsibility for the contract used by retainees and their practices, there is good evidence that confidence and morale is linked to poor employment practice.

As Maslow's hierarchy of need suggests, it is difficult for an individual to fulfil their potential without their basic needs being addressed.[8] Several deaneries had questionnaired their retainees and found a wide range of terms and conditions.[9] Although rare, we all reported finding retainees with no contracts and some who were self-employed. Particular issues for the retainees were no paid study leave, no paid annual leave and no maternity leave; fortunately these instances were rare and we were able to assist them. Some retainees said that after their professional expenses and childcare costs were deducted from their taxed income they did not make a profit, so that working was simply a way to keep their hand in while their children were young.

Deaneries had found different solutions to these problems. In London, the deanery had written to both practices and retainees to tell them the spread of pay and other terms and conditions, so that they were all aware of the variations. Another method was to get retainees to meet up annually and share their experiences. A show of hands at these meetings empowered those with the worst conditions to have the courage to go back to their practices and renegotiate if they were well out of line with their colleagues. It seemed that getting retainees together was a very powerful tool for increasing their confidence around these issues; many had felt very isolated beforehand.

Some deaneries annually met up with their retainees individually. This often enabled those with the worst conditions to speak to their practices and resolve problems. Trent and the London Deaneries have produced handbooks, which clarify many issues, and the guidance was greatly welcomed by practices and retainees. The Eastern Deanery had been told by their retainees that their *Frequently Asked Questions* document had been invaluable.

The dream

The very best conditions based on best practice. What would it look like?

- All retainees to have a modern contract
- Deaneries to questionnaire their retainees
- Annual deanery-wide retainer meetings
- Mentor/tutor from the deanery to help resolve issues about education and the scheme
- Handbook for retainees, with contacts for NHS childcare, tutors, BMA, RCGP, doctor support line, occupational health etc.

Conclusion

We all agreed that this group of GPs was extremely content and grateful to be able to work at times that suited their lives, in quality practices and with educational opportunities that enabled them to continue to develop. Given the current culture of long working hours we felt that it was essential that this scheme continues in order to address the problem of finding suitable employment to retain GPs who are temporarily unable to work more than a limited number of hours for personal or domestic reasons. Our aim is firstly to continue to improve the educational component and working conditions of these GPs so that they retain and improve their skills and confidence, and secondly to be able to offer a choice of career paths to select from when they become ready to return to more full-time general practice.[10]

Using our dream as a way forward, it is encouraging to reflect on the progress that has been made since we left our meeting armed with long 'to do' lists. Great strides have been taken in the last few months, with the Department of Health having announced the creation of a new flexible career scheme, and with a range of improvements in the scheme at local levels – a new web discussion forum for retainees, several new learning sets, away days, handbooks, preparation of an updated retainer scheme contract and plans for both local and national surveys.

References

1 Cooperrider DL and Srivastva S (1987) Appreciative inquiry in organisational life. *Research in Organizational Change and Development.* **1**: 129–69.

2 Department of Health (1999) *GP Retainer Scheme; guidance on the educational aspects of the scheme.* HSC 1999/004. NHS Executive, Leeds.

3 Fox J (1999) A study of non-principals in the Mersey Deanery. In: Educating GP non-principals. *Educ Gen Pract.* **10**: 359–60 (Supplement).

4 Oxenbury J (1999) Appropriate education for non-principals. In: Educating GP non-principals. *Educ Gen Pract.* **10**: 350–2 (Supplement).

5 Viney R and Muller E (2002) Continuing professional development for GP non-principals; but still not enough flour to bake a cake. In: Continuing Professional Development for GP non-principals. *Educ Prim Care.* **13**: 115–16 (Supplement).

6 Woodwark F, Pitts J and Smith F (2002) Responsibilities and preparedness of educational supervisors of GP retainees: a view from both sides. *Educ Prim Care.* **13**: 35–41.

7 Department of Health. *Improving Working Lives.* www.doh.gov.uk/iwl

8 Maslow A (1970) *Motivation and Personality (2e).* Harper and Row, New York.

9 Taylor G (2002) The doctor's retainer scheme in general practice – from service to education? A questionnaire survey. *Educ Prim Care.* **13**: 150–7.

10 Hastie A (2002) An assessment of the GP retainer scheme. *Educ Prim Care.* **13**: 233–8.

Based on a workshop given at the 2002 UKCEA conference. With thanks to the workshop participants Drs Anne Hastie, Iain Cromarty, Jas Bilkhu, Mike Ruscoe, R Weaver.

CHAPTER 16

An educational approach to significant event analysis and risk management in primary care

Paul Bowie and John McKay

Significant event analysis (SEA) is encouraged in general practice as an important method of reflective learning that can contribute to our continuing education and professional development. In addition to its educational potential, SEA may also inform and impact on many other issues of importance to the clinical governance agenda. Improving the quality of healthcare; enhancing patient safety; minimising healthcare risk; and facilitating needs assessment, are just a few of the areas that may potentially benefit from the routine use of SEA by healthcare practitioners.

The SEA technique involves the identification and critical review of individual case studies or events, which have happened in everyday practice and are considered to be 'significant' by those involved. Pringle and colleagues define a significant event as '... any event thought by anyone in the team to be significant in terms of patient care or the conduct of the practice'.[1]

SEA is in effect a qualitative form of retrospective audit, however unlike (quantitative) criterion-based audit, it is a more flexible and probably less taxing technique. In this respect, SEA is able to address a much wider range of issues in less time and without the need for large-scale data collection than conventional audit.

Central to the SEA process is that it involves taking a non-threatening, no-blame approach towards identifying and resolving significant events. Importantly it should be undertaken as a multidisciplinary exercise where openness and the building of trust amongst team members is strongly encouraged for the best results. This is especially so when discussing adverse incidents or potentially sensitive topics that may otherwise have been treated superficially or even ignored altogether in the past.

The success of SEA is highly dependent upon this type of open, self-critical environment being nurtured within a practice team. However it should also be remembered that not every significant event necessarily has a negative connotation. The SEA process actively encourages team members to identify and 'celebrate' those significant events that can highlight and confirm instances of good practice. In reality, however, most significant events, whether clinical or administrative, can be broadly categorised as adverse occurrences, near misses or errors.

SEA and peer review in the West of Scotland Deanery

In the West of Scotland Deanery, all GPs can submit SEA reports of their choice for peer review assessment. To date some 401 SEA reports have been submitted by a total of 219 GPs in the deanery. The reports are submitted in a standard format developed by 20 trained GP SEA assessors. Two randomly chosen assessors from this group independently review a SEA report using a criterion-referenced assessment schedule, which has been developed to ensure that insight into the event is demonstrated, lessons are learnt and change is implemented, where feasible. SEA reports are confidential and anonymous to the assessors. One session of PGEA is awarded for each submission and written educational feedback is given based on any issues raised by the assessors.

The main purpose of this type of approach to SEA is not only to encourage practitioners to identify significant events, but also to perform a structured analyses of the events, rather than just a superficial discussion and an agreement 'to try and improve' or, worse still, just ignore them. In this way the practitioner can gain insight into the highlighted event, learn from it and take appropriate action (where necessary) to avoid or minimise recurrence in the future. The advantage of a peer review system is that it not only adds rigour and an element of quality assurance to the SEA process, but also acts as an educational support and advisory mechanism for those engaged in SEA activity.

The format used for the structured analysis of an event in the deanery revolves around detailed consideration of the following four questions:

1   What happened?
2   Why did it happen?
3   What have we learnt?
4   What have we changed?

An illustrated case study of a typical example of a significant event analysis submitted for peer assessment in the deanery is outlined in the Box below.

Significant event analysis – case study

What happened?
A patient arrived at the reception desk to pick up a prescription for Amitriptyline. He was given the prescription for Amitriptyline dated the previous day, but in addition there was also a prescription for Amitriptyline which had been lying there from the month before and he was also given this prescription. The patient therefore had a large amount of Amitriptyline at home and over the following few days an overdose was taken, with hospital admission and monitoring required.

Why did it happen?
Issues that could be discussed here include the:

- system to identify prescriptions which have not been collected
- system to minimise the quantity of potentially dangerous drugs available to patient and follow-up of patients with significant illness using potentially dangerous drugs
- GP practice prescribing for patient normally reviewed in secondary care.

What are the main learning points?
- There is no foolproof system to stop this patient hoarding medication and subsequently overdosing, however risk can be reduced.
- Change needs to be implemented to put in place a system which regularly checks for 'old' prescriptions and allows action, if necessary, to be taken.

What would you change? Potential solutions:
- named person to remove prescriptions from prescription box after a specified number of days if not collected
- prescription then to be destroyed or prescriber notified
- repeat prescriptions for potentially dangerous drugs to be 'tagged' so that when a new prescription is generated a check can be made that any previous prescription has been uplifted
- prescription may be marked weekly dispense to minimise volume available
- possible increased review of patients on particular medications to assess risk
- discussion with pharmacist, if patient uses the same pharmacy to 'flag up' issues over frequency of dispensing.

SEA: the evidence base

Research

Almost a decade after the concept of significant event analysis was first proposed, the evidence base to support the various claims about its potential benefits is either very limited or non-existent. In addition to the groundbreaking
work undertaken by Bradley[2] and Pringle et al.,[1] the published research base
consists mainly of qualitative studies undertaken recently.[3-7]

SEA research in the West of Scotland Deanery

Recent research into SEA in the deanery has concentrated on studying both the
peer assessment system developed locally and the experiences and opinions of
SEA gained from principals in general practice in Greater Glasgow.

An evaluation of the first 146 SEA reports voluntarily submitted by 84 GPs for
assessment by peer review took place in January 2001.[8] The study concluded
that the documented implementation of change relevant to the significant
event was a highly significant factor in successful peer assessment of submitted
SEA reports. In addition the study findings indicated that a total of 64% of
all submitted SEA reports were considered satisfactory by peer assessment.
Furthermore, only a small proportion of SEA reports undertaken, around 15%,
appear to have been directly influenced by complaints to the practice.

In a further, as yet unpublished, study involving the educational peer assessment of SEA reports, Bowie et al. reported on the personal and professional
characteristics of GPs participating in the system. A total of 126 (6%) GPs in the
region had participated in the peer assessment at this stage of its development
by submitting 237 SEA reports. GP trainers submitted considerably more SEA
reports than other colleagues from training and non-training environments.
A total of 62% of SEAs were peer-reviewed as satisfactory, with GP trainers also
significantly more likely to have their SEA assessed satisfactorily than other colleagues from both training and non-training practices. Being a member of the
RCGP did not appear to influence whether a SEA report was satisfactorily
reviewed by the assessors.

The extent to which SEA is undertaken in general practice is currently
unknown. Anecdotal evidence suggests that around 20% of GPs routinely
participate in this activity.[9] A large cross-sectional study (unpublished) has produced the first quantities survey data on the reported SEA experiences of Greater
Glasgow GPs and their attitudes towards its application. The findings (76%
response rate, 471/617) suggest that up to 60% report undertaking a structured

analysis of a recent significant event that happened in their practices. It is difficult, however, to both quantify the level of SEA activity undertaken and verify the claims that a structured analysis of a significant event actually takes place rather than a general discussion. A minority of respondents report that they were unaware of any recent significant events in practice. A quarter agree that they are uncertain how to properly analyse a significant event and a large minority report difficulty in determining when an event is actually 'significant'. Just under one-third believe SEA can cause problems between staff, while a similar number admit that significant events are often not acted upon in their practices, with one-fifth of respondents reporting that they sometimes avoid dealing with significant events because of the complexity involved.

Further research

There is much still to be learnt about the academic and practical application of the SEA process. In particular the issues of what constitutes 'significance', the understanding of the method and the verification of the outcome all require to be explored. Furthermore, the levels of impact SEA has on actually improving patient care or enhancing risk management are also major issues that require more detailed research.

Issues arising

What is meant by 'significant'?

Pringle and colleagues acknowledge that the broad definition of a significant event provided in his groundbreaking work may cause potential problems with the choice of events to be studied.[1] However, they suggest that a system should be put in place to enable identified significant events to be prioritised by the practice team. In this way the practice can focus on those events that are more likely to stimulate interest and provoke discussion amongst team members.

The appropriateness of this broad definition and the need to prioritise in relation to the types of significant events that GPs may choose to analyse was an issue raised by the group. For example, if a GP on a house visit happens to be bitten by a dog can this be classed as a significant event? Undoubtedly this is a significant event for the unfortunate individual concerned. However, would spending time on a structured analysis of this event necessarily lead to improvements in patient care or a more effective practice organisation?

Educational benefit

Using the above definition of significant event analysis, many practices may routinely choose to analyse significant diagnoses (such as cancer), find that their care has been satisfactory and agree that they have no need to change practice or behaviour in this instance. While this may reassure these practitioners the question remains as to whether other events taking place in the practice would be more usefully discussed and analysed. Indeed previous research has shown that implementing change as part of SEA is more likely to be regarded by peers as educationally satisfactory.[8] Priority, therefore, should perhaps be given to those significant events that not only stimulate discussion and interest amongst the team as Pringle and colleagues advocate, but also to those that can potentially lead to the implementation of change in the practice.

Practice team involvement

The crucial issue in the success of SEA relates to team dynamics. It is essential that the analysis of significant events by the practice team should take place in an environment conducive to open and non-threatening discussion. All team members, from the receptionist to the senior partner, should have equal opportunity to contribute to the SEA agenda. However, it is recognised that certain significant events, particularly those that are purely clinical, need only be analysed by those responsible for the delivery of care and treatment.

SEA: appraisal and mandatory incident reporting

It has been suggested that SEA should be an integral part of the appraisal process involving all GPs. However, several concerns have been noted in relation to the analysis and documentation of significant events that external appraisers may have direct access to, and the associated legal implications. Some GPs may avoid documenting significant events that reflect poorly on themselves or the practice, even though corrective action has clearly taken place. Even more concerning would be if practitioners felt so threatened by external review of their SEA that they then avoided addressing the more serious significant events that have happened. Indeed we already know from the survey of Greater Glasgow GPs mentioned earlier that the vast majority reported their unwillingness to participate in a mandatory incident reporting system, preferring instead a local, voluntary and anonymised system of reporting.

PGEA and SEA

The system used in the west of Scotland appears an effective way to encourage the independent analysis of significant events by offering an educational incentive. Anecdotal evidence from participating GPs suggests that this is a practical, straightforward and worthwhile method of gaining a single PGEA session. The exponential increase in the number of SEA reports received every year since the system started is testament to the popularity of this educational method amongst GPs. The one drawback is that this system is GP-centred, however the possibility exists that this can be adapted for multidisciplinary use.

Conclusion

There is general agreement that promoting SEA through education is a worthwhile activity for GPs given the professional and organisational obligations associated with revalidation and clinical governance. From a peer assessment perspective, further development of the SEA process is required within the practice structure in order to involve the whole primary care team, although this may prove complex. On the research front, clear evidence of the benefits and impact of SEA is still to be adequately demonstrated. However, there is no doubting the attraction and potential of SEA as a technique for quality improvement and risk management.

References

1 Pringle M, Bradley CP, Carmichael CM *et al.* (1995) Significant event auditing: a study of the feasibility and potential of case-based auditing in primary medical care. Royal College of General Practitioners, London.

2 Bradley CP (1992) Turning anecdotes into data – the critical incident technique. *Fam Pract.* **9**: 98–103.

3 Westcott R, Sweeney G and Stead J (2000) Significant event audit in practice: a preliminary study. *Fam Pract.* **17**: 173–9.

4 Sweeney G, Westcott R and Stead J (2000) The benefits of significant event audit in primary care: a case study. *J Clin Gov.* **8**: 128–34.

5 Mitchell G and Pachmajer U (2001) Significant event audit as a means of defining the value of general practice to a health system: a proposal. *Eur J Gen Pract.* **7**: 115–17.

6 Wilkes D and Mills K (2001) Using the significant event audit model and patient interviews in assessing the quality of care. *J Clin Gov.* **9**: 13–19.

7 Fox M, Sweeney G, Howells C *et al.* (2001) Significant event audit in prison healthcare: changing a culture for clinical governance – a qualitative study. *J Clin Gov.* **9**: 123–8.

8 McKay J, Bowie P and Lough M (2002) Evaluating significant event analyses: implementing change is a measure of success. *Educ Prim Care* (In press).

9 Wilson T, Smith F and Lakhani M (2002) Patient safety in primary healthcare – an overview of current developments in risk management and implications for clinical governance. *J Clin Gov.* **10**: 25–30.

Based on a workshop given at the 2002 UKCEA conference. With thanks to the workshop participants Drs Maureen Crawford, Richard Flew, Peter Havelock, Dr Vish Kini, Barry Lewis and Alan Rogers.

CHAPTER 17

Underperforming doctors and the deanery role

Reed Bowden

Medical educationalists at all levels are increasingly involved in procedures to assess and assist colleagues who are struggling or persistently underperforming in their practices. The extent to which dcaneries should be involved in the management of underperformance has been repeatedly aired in the medical education literature and was an issue of prime concern at the 2002 UKCEA conference. It is therefore timely to review the present position and likely direction of travel.

In 1997 the GMC introduced procedures under a new committee, the Committee on Professional Performance (CPP), to investigate doctors whose practice put their patients at unacceptable risk. The report produced by the School of Health and Related Research, University of Sheffield (ScHARR) provided the backdrop,[1] the work of Southgate provided the means of assessment,[2] and the law underpinned the whole exercise. At the same time health authorities were urged to introduce assessment procedures for doctors whose work was below an acceptable standard but not poor enough to be drawn to the attention of the GMC, and who were thought to be amenable to improvement with local help. Some health authorities responded to the call immediately, others tarried, but local support groups (LSGs) or their equivalents under other titles (these days the term performance panel is often used) eventually appeared everywhere. In some areas the task was devolved to PCOs, usually to the chairs of their clinical governance subcommittees, who might call on general practice tutors to help. Now that health authorities are evolving into strategic health authorities the responsibility for this work will devolve to PCTs, which will need to allot funds and find the people to make it work. The operative date for the system to be in place is 1 October 2002.

The essential difference between local and GMC procedures is that the local system is based in regulation rather than law, and cannot of itself put the doctor's registration at risk.

There is no generally-agreed definition of persistent underperformance, but typically a LSG would be asked to consider doctors who have generated three complaints or more in two years, or where there are misgivings about their performance arising from several different sources (the concept of triangulation). Sometimes evidence comes from employed or attached staff, or from partners. On other occasions colleagues such as local consultants might report inappropriate, excessive or poorly documented referrals. Suspicions about performance are often backed up by indirect evidence from performance indicators. Prescribing advisers may note bizarre prescribing habits from PACT figures. Other statistics held by health authorities, such as PGEA attendance or staff turnover, may deviate widely from the mean. Wherever the evidence comes from, it must be rigorous and attested. Vague accusations and rumours will not do.

The committee must decide whether to seek an assessment visit, to refer to the GMC, or to wait and see; eventually it will also now have the option of referral to the NCAA. If, in the LSG's judgement, there should be an assessment visit, the usual course is to arrange for a subgroup (sometimes called an assessment and action panel) to visit the doctor at his or her place of work. The subgroup may be one person, charged with making an educational assessment, or preferably a group comprising a health authority primary care development officer, a local medical committee (LMC) member and an educationalist, perhaps with a lay assessor in addition. The benefit of sending a larger group is that the difficulties in which these doctors find themselves are seldom a simple matter of ongoing education, but may involve poor premises, ill-health, partner and team problems, excessive workload and many other factors. The prime aim of the team is to ensure reasonable patient safety. The fixed points by which to steer are contained in the GMC booklets *Good Medical Practice*[3] and *Maintaining Good Medical Practice*.[4] As far as GPs are concerned, the advice in these pamphlets is refined and expanded in *Good Medical Practice for General Practitioners* put out jointly by the General Practitioners' Committee of the BMA and the RCGP.[5] One point that must be emphasised is that the basis of local assessment is meant to be help and not censure. Some deaneries are content to send educationalists to make assessments alone, unsupported by colleagues from the LMC, PCT or health authority. There is therefore a risk of missing non-educational causes for poor performance, and also a theoretical risk that legal action arising from the assessment could have to be answered by the deanery representative alone.

There is another group of clients besides those coming directly from LSGs, which directors (or deans) must consider. These are doctors who have been through formal GMC procedures, and are then referred back to deaneries with special educational requirements during a period of conditional registration. They form a fascinating group. Not all come from the CPP. Some come from the health committee, often after mental illness or problems to do with substance abuse. Health committee referees, and only these, do not have to fund their remedial supervision; deaneries must find the money to pay trainers for them. A few are referred from the professional conduct committee. The instructions that accompany this group can show detachment from reality on the part of the GMC, or perhaps wry humour. Two recent examples from London will make the point. One doctor who had sold NHS prescriptions for addictive drugs to addicts came with instructions to 'revise his knowledge of prescribing'. Another, whose proclivity was to allow his hands to wander towards intimate areas of his female patients, was told to 'improve his communication skills'. Leaving aside these rarities, most GMC clients will arrive from the CPP. There will be a set of instructions, the committee's 'determination' as it is known, which lists the headings in *Good Medical Practice*[3] where deficiencies have been shown, based on a mass of evidence, the most important being the results of the assessors' visit to the doctor's practice and the scores in the formal tests. The scores are sent to the doctor himself, and he will normally make them available to the associate director or dean (AD) advising him. Several problems arise for the dean at this point. First, the list of deficiencies is often so long that remediation may amount to complete retraining. Next, the restrictions on the doctor's practice usually include attachment to an approved trainer, and further restrictions mean that no form of independent practice is possible; this makes the doctor difficult to place. Trainers, understandably, want to train young doctors keen to enter general practice, not mature doctors in difficulties. From the client's point of view a new and unwelcome burden is laid on them. They receive no pay while retraining, and there is no money available from the GMC or the deanery for their trainer. This means they must negotiate payment with the trainer, and this will come from their own pocket. This double whammy often coincides with heavy outgoings, such as the university costs of children, and mortgage expenses. It could be argued that erasure would be kinder for some, and providing funds would be a good investment in others, particularly when many years' more service to the NHS might be anticipated, and when in many cases the original costs of medical training were borne by another country.

The cost of remedial education for the locally identified doctors, to whom we shall now return, is much less, and easier to bear, as these doctors will be carrying on with their work in their own practices, albeit with considerable educational supervision.

There is some impatience with the GMC, both with the delays that can beset assessment, and also with the unrealistic expectations of deanery help expressed in the conditions attached to some doctors' registration after performance hearings. It is hoped that COGPED will take a lead in negotiating to improve this.

As mentioned above, doctors who give cause for concern at LSG level are, by arrangement and with consent, visited at their practice, if they have one. The question then arises of how the assessment should proceed, and how the visiting subgroup might divide up their work. A typical visit might include an interview with the doctor to present the group's bona fides and to enquire tactfully about any health or personality factors that may apply. Then the AD would check note-keeping skills, discuss the management of one or two patients prompted by the notes, look at the repeat prescribing system if any, and check the complaints book. Meanwhile other team members may look at the premises, including health and safety issues, interview members of staff, and check the waiting room, doctor accessibility, and clinics. In the writer's opinion the initial assessment should occupy the group for no more than half a day, the equivalent of 15 or 16 person-hours of input. This means that an assessment toolkit such as the RCGP/St Paul document, though worthy, is too unwieldy for routine use, though its summary may be found helpful.[6]

The initial assessment is presented to the doctor as a report, which he is invited to check for factual accuracy. When that is done the report can then be re-presented as a plan for action, with each area for remediation given a timescale over which improvements should take place. Subsequent visits, which may not be by the whole group, are made to check that progress is occurring. Education is always part of the plan of action. Often the only postgraduate education that the doctor has taken part in is the local PGEA programme, which has been accepted uncritically and with no attempt at a personal educational needs assessment. Indeed, concepts like 'needs assessment', and many of the other terms which are the small change of conversation between people who accept the importance of continuing education, may be quite new to many of these doctors. Audit activity, PUNs and DENs,[7] critical event analysis[8] and many other concepts and requirements may be received blankly. To begin to turn this around may require help from various quarters, including personal commitment from an educationalist or mentor, the help of the GP tutor, and input from the PCT with protocols and formularies. A new approach which has just been piloted by the London Deanery is to offer a week's course, concentrating on areas where a lot of remedial work is often needed, such as consultation skills and prescribing. The week also includes a simulated surgery, similar to the one offered by the RCGP as an alternative to video analysis of consultation skills,[9] followed by confidential feedback of results and individual advice from an examiner.

All this activity presents problems for deaneries although the extent of deanery involvement with these doctors varies greatly around the country. In some areas deans deny that a problem exists. Others are heavily involved in assessment or remediation, or both. How much of this work should they take on? Is it right to be involved both with assessing underperformers and recommending and supervising the educational part of their remediation? Some answers are beginning to emerge.

Most deans and directors have accepted that to have ADs sitting as members of LSGs is a sensible and legitimate use of deanery resources, but assessments and follow-ups arising from LSG work are a duty too far. This work can mean finding extra sessions of AD time. Some health authorities have decided to fund these additional sessions. Others prefer to pay what amounts to piecework rates for deans or freelance educationalists to help with each case. It seems sensible to keep assessment and remediation separate if possible, but the volume of work is likely to mean that some people will take part in both.

The NCAA came into existence on 1 April 2001, as promised in the document *Supporting Doctors, Protecting Patients*,[10] and in the wake of a number of infamous cases of poor performance. The follow-up document *Assuring the Quality of Medical Practice*[11] sets out more about it. In the autumn of 2001 it began to receive pilot referrals about doctors whose performance needed attention, and is currently working through a group of them, with the hope that a managed system of assessment sufficient to cope with full demand will be in place by the end of 2003. It appears that the NCAA will have some duties as a triage organisation, and some as an investigative one. Though it will use trained assessors under its own banner, both lay and medical, the workload will require existing LSG teams to carry on with their work as well. There is one function which the NCAA could take on, and which would satisfy many who are concerned at the lack of validated and approved assessment tools for LSG teams, and that is that the NCAA's working groups might be prepared to approve a selection of such tools so that our clients can be assured of even-handed treatment throughout the country. There is a promise of some funding for locums when NCAA clients need them. There are also hopes that the NCAA will monitor outcomes.

As we approach revalidation, it may be appropriate to consider where, if anywhere, this will link with underperformance.[12] Although the details of the revalidation package are still not completely clear, even though the system is scheduled to begin in April 2002, we know that annual appraisal will be part of it. Until recently it was axiomatic that the appraisers would not act as snoopers for underperformance, except that an immediate and severe danger to patients would oblige any of us to blow the whistle. That apart, the two processes were to be quite separate. It seems now that this decision may have been reversed. Appraisal will merge into performance management, and failure to recommend revalidation will mean automatic referral to the GMC. This may well encourage doctors approaching revalidation and who have the insight to be concerned about their own performance to retire gracefully at this time. Hopefully the revalidation process might eventually cover most of the work at present undertaken with respect to underperformance so that deaneries could use their educational expertise in other fields.

References

1   Rotherham G, Martin D, Joesbury H *et al.* (1997) *Measures to Assist General Practitioners whose Performance Gives Cause for Concern.* University of Sheffield, Sheffield.

2   Southgate L (ed.) (2001) The GMC'S performance procedures: a study of their implementation and impact. *Medical Education.* **35**(Supplement 1).

3 GMC (2001) *Good Medical Practice* (3e). GMC, London.

4 GMC (1998) *Maintaining Good Medical Practice*. GMC, London.

5 RCGP (2000) *Good Medical Practice for General Practitioners*. RCGP, London.

6 RCGP (2001) *Summary Document: toolkit for managing general practitioners whose performance gives concern*. RCGP, London.

7 Eve R (2000) Learning with PUNs and DENs – a method for determining the educational needs and the evaluation of its use in primary care. *Educ Gen Pract.* **11**: 73–9.

8 Pringle M and Bradley C (1994) Significant event auditing: a user's guide. *Audit Trends.* **2**: 20–3.

9 Burrows P and Bingham L (1999) The simulated surgery – an alternative to video submission for the consulting skills component of the MRCGP examination: the first year's experience. *Br J Gen Pract.* **49**: 269–72.

10 Department of Health (1999) *Supporting Doctors, Protecting Patients*. Department of Health, London.

11 Department of Health (2001) *Assuring the Quality of Medical Practice*. Department of Health, London.

12 (www.gmc-uk.org/revalidation)

Based on a workshop discussion at the 2002 UKCEA conference and a recent review article from Education for Primary Care *(Bowden R, The under performing doctor, 13: 223–7) refashioned here by kind permission of the Editor.*

CHAPTER 18

The assessment of underperformance – towards a toolkit for local use

John Schofield

The problem of assessing the performance of doctors is clearly taxing many of us in the UK. At the 2002 UKCEA conference the subject generated a great deal of useful discussion on the present state of play and what departments of postgraduate GP education can hope for in the future. I have tried to set out both the basis on which our work in these departments is founded, and the practical applications of particular assessment tools.

Most of the principles underpinning the assessment of underperformance were brought together by the GMC in *Good Medical Practice*[1] with much of the work based research carried out in Sheffield by ScHARR.[2] The concept of some standard tools that are recognised and validated is highly appealing as most of us in educational management feel anxious about exactly what our position is, where the boundaries to our responsibility lie and how we stand legally. It may well be that the NCAA will help to address these concerns in the near future.[3]

There are endless possibilities as to how help might be extended to underperforming doctors, but quite how best this can be done, and by whom, remains a developing field. The costs involved in providing high quality remedial training also pose a dilemma.

This chapter is based on a workshop discussion held at the 2002 UKCEA conference and the questions that were addressed in that workshop are considered here, namely:

- Are toolkits for assessing performance being used?
- If so, please let's share them.
- Is there a place for a national toolkit or is local development preferable?
- Are summative assessment tools applicable to this group of doctors?

- How do we measure poor performance in the context of everyday general practice?
- Can the performance of the doctors be separated from the context of the practice?
- How can we bring all this together?

Stakeholders

In considering the assessment of underperformance it is important to identify the main stakeholders. The following groups are suggested.

- Patients – clearly the safety and well-being of patients is paramount.
- Doctors – there was general agreement that any process should be seen as fair and open. They should be treated equitably.
- The profession – the recent well-publicised cases not only affect the particular doctors but also reflect on the rest of the profession, making relationships with patients more difficult.
- Society – the rest of the communities besides the patient need to feel that proper procedures are in place to deal effectively with problems.
- Funding sources – those paying the bill need to be reassured that good quality work is being done on their behalf. There also should be clear agreement as to how remedial work is to be funded so as to reduce future mistakes.

In other words, the situation is complex and dynamic with multiple stakeholders and divergent pathways of responsibility. Further evidence to support this view is apparent when we consider the agencies to which underperforming GPs are required to relate.

Agencies relating to underperforming GPs

Many and various public and professional bodies are concerned with an underperforming GP either in a regulatory or supportive role. A diagrammatic summary of these relationships is presented below (*see* Figure 18.1) and although this is not entirely comprehensive, it does give some idea of the 'quadruple jeopardy' that the underperforming GP may be exposed to.

Where does the GP educationalist fit into this oppressive structure? It is generally agreed that our role should be to help with assessing the competence of the doctor, providing an educational prescription and trying to identify opportunities for education appropriate to the situation. This role is explored in depth

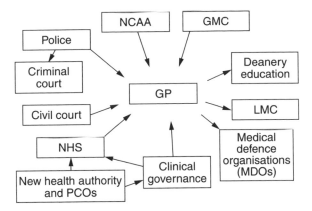

Figure 18.1 Relationships between agencies involved with underperforming GPs.

in Reed Bowden's chapter elsewhere in this book, 'Underperforming doctors and the deanery role' (Chapter 17).

In reality the boundaries of an educationalist's role can become very blurred. The great advantage that we have is that we actually have no power to compel the referred doctor to participate and thus the majority of these GPs are really quite keen to have our help.

A structure for assessment

The usual process for assessing the underperforming doctor is outlined in Figure 18.2.

Considerable anxiety is engendered by some of the stages of this process, in particular the decisions around 'signing off' or discharging the underperforming doctor from remedial care. If further problems arise, where does liability and responsibility lie? The other major area of concern is how long a doctor should be allowed to go round and round the assessment–remediation cycle without an outcome being finally decided. Clearly if no progress is being made then referral on to the GMC would be necessary at some point. Again some statement or agreement of national standards would be extremely helpful.

From discussions at the UKCEA conference, remedial action is being implemented in different ways in different areas of the country. Quite often the doctors concerned are in need of intensive help or retraining in particular skills such as 'the consultation'. It is not always easy to find suitable training services, which address the particular needs, and these may be very labour intensive and expensive to provide.

Around the country, the consensus view appears to be that the doctor concerned should fund remediation him or herself. On occasion some outside

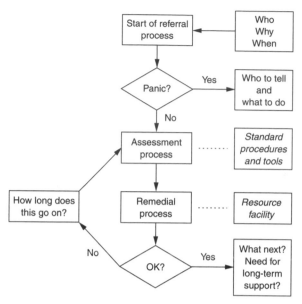

Figure 18.2   The usual process for assessing the underperforming doctor.

funding has been provided by health authorities or PCTs who wish to see the quality of the practices in their areas improved. In the context of a severe GP shortage it may well be cost-effective to try to support a GP through this process if there is a reasonable prospect of success.

A standard bank of assessment tools and processes – ideally NCAA-accredited – is eagerly awaited. There is promising progress in this area as the GMC is shortly to produce a raft of standardised methods for appraising doctors[4] and ScHARR has published a comprehensive document on the appraisal of GPs.[5]

The assessment process

The view from the deaneries is that a typical assessment team should consist of:

- an organisational manager – PCT/health authority
- an educationalist – deanery
- a doctor's friend – LMC
- a practice team person – nurse/practice manager
- a lay person – to give a patient's perspective.

In such a stressed and often highly charged situation, such widespread representation is very important. In addition, the inclusion of a layperson, especially someone familiar with the area, helps to give context and perspective to the assessment. Having a number of people with differing specialities also allows for triangulation – a view from several angles – and if they assess separately, at least initially, then the reliability of the assessment is enhanced.

It is important to separate out problems that relate directly to the doctor and those that are outside his or her control. For instance services may not be provided appropriately because suitable premises or staff are not available. To this end, a team member with HR training can be invaluable.

LMC and/or health authority/PCT representation is especially important as in many cases, the problem may be linked to the health of the doctor concerned. In these circumstances these agencies may well be able to facilitate suitable sick leave and cover arrangements.

Assessment tools and toolkits

As far as existing assessment tools are concerned, most refer directly to the GMC's *Good Medical Practice* which spells out in detail the roles and responsibilities of doctors.[1] Interestingly, prior to the publication of that document, the GMC had always emphasised what a doctor should not do. The choice of assessment tool of course depends on the purposes for which it is to be put, circumstances in which it is to be used and the person using the tool.

From a management point of view, the Rotherham assessment tools can be very useful.[2] These give an overview of the structure and function of a practice. Immunisation rates, targets achieved, PACT figures, the numbers of appropriate staff (practice nurses, receptionists, practice manager) help to build a picture together with the condition and facilities of the premises. A joint visit with PCT or health authority can therefore be used to accelerate the improvement of buildings or to facilitate the recruitment of additional staff. Thus the visit, even though it probably appears very threatening to the doctor, may in itself have positive outcomes.

The St Paul's toolkit, which can be downloaded from the internet, was one freely available resource which has been found to be useful as a starting point.[6]

To assess the doctor's clinical skills we are starting to see some tools that can readily be used. Many of these are based on the well-tried areas for summative assessment[7] and the RCGP exam.[8] In many ways the summative assessment level is more appropriate as this was originally set at 'minimal competence' although has now moved to 'suitable for independent practice'. Agreement has recently been reached that doctors can be entered into the summative assessment test system with a unique identifier thus allowing access to MCQs, EMQs, video consultation analysis, simulated surgeries, and audit. Indeed audit is a common method of assessing a doctor's ability to present his/her work.

Many of us have also used the Phased Evaluation Programme-Compact Discs (PEP-CDs) from Scotland,[9] which give an objective assessment of clinical knowledge.

The familiar vocational training methods of sitting in with a doctor or analysing a video of consultations can also be very informative. It is useful to have some structure prepared beforehand to make notes of the consultations and the marking schedules used for summative assessment, or the MRCGP – perhaps with one or two adjustments – can be used. Even where there have been problems with making a video in the practice it has been found possible to obtain agreement to carry out an audio recording instead.

A PDP and practice professional development plan are very helpful in assessment. There are many off the shelf proformas available, for instance the *Update PDP* which can be downloaded.[10] PDPs also encourage reflective practice and may link in with such formalised methods as PUNs and DENs[11] and significant event analysis.

Some of the most challenging areas are with doctors who have strange personalities or are very angry. Help might be sought from a HR specialist or occupational psychologist in these circumstances.

Conclusions

The subjects of 'performance' and 'what's a good doctor' continue to exercise both the medical and the lay press. The editorial by Wilson and Haslam in the *British Journal of General Practice* sets out clearly many of the problems and dilemmas.[12] Recently the *British Medical Journal* devoted a whole edition to the concept of the 'good doctor'.[13] Naturally how we assess performance and what tools and measures we use depends on what perspective we are coming from.

Like most groups, GPs come with a whole variety of attributes, some of which are measurable and some not. There is also a spectrum of ability and competencies with no easy or clear cut-off point to judge doctors by. Using a variety of tools, which cover the requirements of the major stakeholders, gives a feel for both the breadth and depth of any problems. A longitudinal assessment over several months also helps to clarify whether there is potential for improvement and may well be seen to be a fairer process, if challenged. At the time of the 2002 UKCEA conference we find ourselves with many theoretical structures for assessment. The next step is to try and put some meat on the tools available by using them in the real world and feeding back on our experience of their applicability. The learning process is only just beginning.

References

1 The General Medical Council (1997) *Good Medical Practice*. GMC: (www.gmc-uk.org)

2 Rotherham G, Martin D, Joesbury H *et al.* (1997) *Measures to Assist GPs Whose Performance Gives Cause for Concern*. (www.shef.ac.uk/~scharr)

3   National Clinical Assessment Authority. (www.ncaa.nhs.uk)

4   The General Medical Council. *Appraisal and Revalidation*. (www.appraisals.nhs.uk)

5   Martin D, Harrison P, Joesbury H *et al*. (2001) *Appraisal for GPs*. (www.shef.ac.uk/~scharr)

6   Royal College of General Practitioners. *Toolkit for Managing GPs whose Performance gives Concern*. (www.rcgp.org.uk/rcgp/quality_unit/toolkit/index.asp)

7   The National Office of Summative Assessment. (www.nosa.org.uk)

8   Royal College of General Practitioners. *The MRCGP Examination*. (www.rcgp.org.uk/rcgp/exam/index.asp)

9   Royal College of General Practitioners Scotland (2000) *PEP-2000*. (www.rcgp.org.uk/rcgp/faculties/scotcoun/pepcd/)

10 Update (2001) *Personal Development Plan*. (www.doctorupdate.net/du_education/du_e-ducation.asp)

11 Eve R (2000) Learning with PUNs and DENs – a method of determining educational needs and the evaluation of its use in primary care. *Educ General Pract*. **11**: 73–9. (eve97@msn.com)

12 Wilson T and Haslam D (2002) Managing alleged performance problems – are we ready? *Br J Gen Pract*. **482**: 707–8.

13 Hurwitz B and Vass A (2002) What's a good doctor and how do you make one? *BMJ*. **325**: 667–8.

Based on a workshop given at the 2002 UKCEA conference. With thanks to the workshop participants; Drs Adrian Ball, Jas Bilku, Terry Bradley, Andrew Craven, Agnes McKnight, Martin Rowan-Robinson, Kevin Hill.

CHAPTER 19

New directions for general practice education

Tim Swanwick and Neil Jackson

General practice is changing at an unprecedented pace. Indeed general practice must change, but general practice, we are reassured, will remain central to the delivery of patient care in the United Kingdom.

The personal and continuous service provided by Auden's 'endomorph with gentle hands'[1] is no longer an acceptable model for the delivery of primary care in the twenty-first century. It is not acceptable to a public that demands rapid, 24-hour, access to care. Neither is it acceptable to a generation of young doctors who wish to balance their home and professional lives more successfully, and healthily, than their predecessors. The ramifications of such a paradigm shift are wide-ranging. GPs will need to become more integrated into teams, as opposed to assuming a main provider role. Practices will find themselves unable to provide all aspects of the new primary care, and this will necessitate sharing of provision across surgery sites. Service changes, as a result, will need to be reflected in a new contract, specifically tailored to the needs of local populations, rather than clumsily and inappropriately applied across the whole country. Remuneration as a result will become more closely linked with the needs of populations, monitored by a raft of quality and service indicators.

In other words, there is an urgent need to modernise and redesign what we know as general practice, and to increase capacity and productivity by innovative, inter-disciplinary collaborative working.

All these proposed developments must however be considered in the context of falling morale, the increasingly destabilising effect of constant change, and what we can euphemistically term the 'recruitment challenge'. The need to recruit and retain is acutely felt, particularly in the large conurbations and isolated rural areas. The NHS Plan promises 2000 more GPs working in the UK by 2004 with further increases in consultant and GP numbers over the succeeding three years.[2] There are also pledges to increase numbers in nursing by 20 000 by 2006 and to expand healthcare assistant numbers and mental health workers. As we saw earlier in this book, deaneries are working hard to expand training capacity in addition to rolling out new initiatives such as the flexible career and GP returner schemes; there are also projects in progress up and down the country around international recruitment – Spanish, French and German doctors among others – and mobilising the refugee doctor workforce. Whether at the end of the day these initiatives will result in net workforce gains remains to be seen.

Three major pieces of government policy will radically restructure education and training for the future GP workforce namely:

- the Postgraduate Medical Education and Training Board (PMETB)
- the SHO review
- the new GP contract.

The Postgraduate Medical Education and Training Board

Following the dissemination of a policy statement in 2001, the *General Medical Practice and Specialist Medical Education, Training and Qualifications Order 2003* was published for consultation until January 2003.[3] Legislation is planned to create the PMETB by October 2003, which will have representation from the Royal Medical Colleges, the PG deaneries, doctors in training and doctors delivering training, and the GMC, as well as NHS management and patient representation.

The PMETB will have responsibility for the:

- supervision, development and promotion of education and PG training
- approval of curricula and the setting of standards
- approval of training programmes in postgraduate medical education
- quality assurance of their delivery including recruitment and assessment procedures and development of educational supervisors
- setting and maintenance of standards required for entry to the specialist and new general practice registers
- the issuing of certificates of completion of training
- the assessment of equivalence.

The board will work closely with the Royal Colleges and deaneries, with the lofty intention of ensuring that 'all interests are aligned and represented in the arrangements for PG medical education' whilst aiming to 'consolidate and strengthen the position of the medical Royal Colleges and faculties as essential elements of the education and training process'.[4]

In addition to the PMETB itself, there will be two statutory committees; the Training Committee and the Assessment Committee. The order also facilitatively permits the introduction of improvements in medical education and training without the need for cumbersome legislative change.

The PMETB, through the Assessment Committee, will ensure that effective assessment systems are in place and will ask each college to report on the purpose of its examination, the determination of its content, the development of its test methods, standard setting, the selection and training of examiners, feedback to candidates and the result of appeals and legal challenges. Eventually the board will be responsible for approving programmes of assessment against specific criteria.

For general practice, all this means the demise of the JCPTGP as we know it and perhaps a more meaningful future relationship between the deaneries and the RCGP. It is also clear that the general practice education and training community will need to provide the board with a clear competence-based curriculum against which we must be set an appropriate and relevant professional assessment framework. If nothing else, at least here we have an opportunity to rationalise the assessment burden on our registrars.

The SHO review

Unfinished Business, the SHO review or the Donaldson report, finally appeared in the autumn of 2002.[5] It is a document with huge implications and will affect the training and assessment of every doctor in the UK.

Unfinished Business makes the case for the reform of the SHO grade, citing poor job structure, poorly planned training and an increasing workload. Poor selection and appointment procedures are said to be widespread, and clinical and educational supervision inadequate. There are limited flexible training opportunities, and the grade does not cater for the needs of overseas graduate doctors. On top of all this, *Unfinished Business* also calls for a reform of all Royal College examinations.

In making its recommendations *Unfinished Business* posits five principles, namely that:

- all training should be programme-based, and not just linked to time in service
- there should be an initial broad-based training for all doctors
- individual programmes should be made available for doctors with specific needs
- all programmes should be time-bounded
- movement in and out of training programmes should be easier.

Specific recommendations in relation to general practice include a two year foundation programme which might entail several months in general practice for all doctors. SHOs would then enter one of eight basic specialist training programmes, of which one would be the discipline of general practice. Importantly, training **for** general practice is to take place on top of any training undertaken, during the foundation programme, **in** general practice. Whatever the final structures agreed, deaneries will have their work cut out over the next few years in a redesign of GP training that is unparalleled in general practice since the inception of vocational training in the early 1970s.

Initial consultation over, details of where *Unfinished Business* might take us next is due early in 2003, but it is clear that in avoiding the mistakes made as a result of the hasty introduction of the Calman reforms, change will be a lengthy and drawn out process.

The new GP contract

The new GP contract has been hotly debated and will be voted on by the profession in the Spring of 2003.[6] There are implications in the contract for training and professional development but very little specific mention of education itself.

There are three cornerstones to the contract. Firstly, the contract will be between practice and the PCT, not the GP and the health authority as was formerly the case. As a consequence, the patient list will be held by the practice, not the individual practitioner. Lastly, responsibility for out-of-hours care will fall on the PCT.

Funding will be allocated through PCTs who will receive a unified budget with spending floors in certain areas taking into account three main factors: the range of services provided, the size and demographics of the practice list and the quality of the services as defined by the achievement of certain quality benchmarks.

Primary care services will be delivered in three tiers and practices may choose, and be remunerated, at a specific level namely:

- **essential services**
  the treatment of patients who present as ill and the general management of the dying
- **additional services**
  preventative health measures e.g. vaccinations
- **enhanced services**
  the provision of services in response to national or local pressures e.g. anticoagulation clinics, endoscopy, medical supervision of care homes.

In an attempt to encourage best practice there will be a number of 'quality frameworks' for primary care which will make up a considerable proportion of practice income. The 'quality frameworks' will comprise three main elements:

- **clinical standards**
  related to national and local priorities and determined by the evidence base available for the condition
- **organisational standards**
  related to areas such as HR practices, health and safety, information technology, clinical governance, appraisal and prescribing
- **patient experience**
  determined by the reported views of patients on such areas as doctors' communication skills.

It is clear from the structure of the contract that motivated GPs are being offered considerable incentives. There will inevitably be large-scale organisational changes in localities, and PCTs, assisted by the future development of 'GPs with Special Interests',[7] will begin to develop cross-practice services and economies of scale.

The implications of the new contract for education and training are profound and these wide-reaching reforms pose the question 'what sort of general practice are we training doctors for?'. There are also issues around where the training takes place, whether it should be uni-professional or inter-disciplinary, the arrangements that will surround continuing professional development and many minor questions such as whether out-of-hours experience continues to be a training prerequisite. The new GP contract takes us a long way down the road towards Dr Marie Campkin's parody[8] of Auden's 'partridge plump' family doctor:

> *Give me a doctor, underweight,*
> *Computerised and up-to-date,*
> *A businessman who understands*
> *Accountancy and target bands,*
> *Who demonstrates sincere devotion*
> *To audit and to health promotion –*
> *But when my outlook's for the worse*
> *Refers me to the practice nurse.*

Conclusion

It looks clear then, or as clear as anything ever does look in this perpetually changing National Health Service, that deaneries are here to stay. Implementing the SHO review, whilst responding to the demands of a governmentally accountable PMETB, will be quite a task and will require the assistance of the robust structures and educational networks that currently only the deaneries can provide. It is however a task made all the more difficult by the rapidly evolving nature of primary care and the fundamental issues raised by the introduction of a new GP contract. Deaneries will have to look to their own organisational structures and examine whether they are fit for this new purpose. There is a need for clear and effective leadership, co-ordinated strategic planning and the effective deployment of resources. Deaneries must also forge or strengthen existing relationships and begin to work in collaborative partnership with emergent organisations ranging from PCTs, through the WDCs and strategic health authorities to new national bodies such as the NCAA.

The world of PG general practice education in the NHS is complex and dynamic, and our challenge is to manage that complexity today, while planning effectively for tomorrow. Departmental policy initiatives continue to rain down at an impressive rate but the general direction of travel is becoming gradually clearer. We must move towards a new model of primary care, supported by well structured competency-based training linked to timely and relevant assessment programmes. We must offer appropriate educational support, not only for doctors in training, but also doctors in transition and doctors in established practice. And we must respond to the public, to whom we are ultimately accountable, by ensuring the effective regulation and monitoring of medical practice and the involvement of patients at all levels of primary care.

References

1 Auden WH (1994) Give me a doctor, partridge-plump. In: J Gross (ed.) *The Oxford Book of Comic Verse*. Oxford University Press, Oxford.

2 Department of Health (2000) *The NHS Plan*. (www.nhs.uk/nationalplan/nhsplan.htm)

3 Department of Health. *The General Medical Practice and Specialist Medical Education, Training and Qualifications Order 2003*. (www.doh.gov.uk/medicaltrainingintheuk/pmetborder. htm)

4 Department of Health (2001) *The Postgraduate Medical Education and Training Board: Statement on Policy*. (www.doh.gov.uk/medicaltrainingintheuk/pmetbpolicy.pdf)

5 Department of Health (2002) *Unfinished Business*. (www.doh.gov.uk/shoconsult/ubho _1.htm)

6 Royal College of General Practitioners (2002) *Summary of the Draft New GP Contract*. (www.rcgp.org/rcgp/information/publications/summaries/summary02/rcs0003.asp)

7 Royal College of General Practitioners (2002) *Frameworks for GPs with Special Interests (GPSIs)*. (www.rcgp.org.uk/rcgp/corporate/framework_gpsis.asp)

8 Campkin M (2002) Quoted by Field S *The Changing Face of GP Education and Training in the UK*. (www.rcgp.org.uk/rcgp/education/presentations/changing_face/tsld006.htm)

Index